Update on Fibro-Cartilaginous Disease

Editor

MICHAEL H. THEODOULOU

CLINICS IN PODIATRIC MEDICINE AND SURGERY

www.podiatric.theclinics.com

Consulting Editor
THOMAS J. CHANG

July 2022 • Volume 39 • Number 3

ELSEVIER

1600 John F. Kennedy Boulevard • Suite 1800 • Philadelphia, Pennsylvania, 19103-2899

http://www.theclinics.com

CLINICS IN PODIATRIC MEDICINE AND SURGERY Volume 39, Number 3
July 2022 ISSN 0891-8422, ISBN-13: 978-0-323-91963-0

Editor: Megan Ashdown
Developmental Editor: Diana Grace Ang

Clinics in Podiatric Medicine and Surgery (ISSN 0891-8422) is published quarterly by Elsevier Inc., 360 Park Avenue South, New York, NY 10010-1710. Months of issue are January, April, July, and October. Business and Editorial Offices: 1600 John F. Kennedy Blvd., Ste. 1800, Philadelphia, PA 19103-2899. Customer Service Office: 3251 Riverport Lane, Maryland Heights, MO 63043. Periodicals postage paid at New York, NY and additional mailing offices. Subscription prices are $319.00 per year for US individuals, $773.00 per year for US institutions, $100.00 per year for US students and residents, $393.00 per year for Canadian individuals, $796.00 for Canadian institutions, $476.00 for international individuals, $796.00 per year for international institutions, $100.00 per year for Canadian students/residents, and $220.00 per year for foreign students/residents. To receive student/resident rate, orders must be accompanied by name of affiliated institution, date of term, and the *signature* of program/residency coordinator on institution letterhead. Orders will be billed at individual rate until proof of status is received. Foreign air speed delivery is included in all *Clinics* subscription prices. All prices are subject to change without notice. POSTMASTER: Send address changes to *Clinics in Podiatric Medicine and Surgery*, Elsevier Health Sciences Division, Subscription Customer Service, 3251 Riverport Lane, Maryland Heights, MO 63043. **Customer Service: 1-800-654-2452 (US). From outside of the US, call 314-447-8871. Fax: 314-447-8029. E-mail: JournalsCustomerService-usa@elsevier.com (for print support); JournalsOnlineSupport-usa@elsevier.com (for online support).**

Reprints. For copies of 100 or more of articles in this publication, please contact the Commercial Reprints Department, Elsevier Inc., 360 Park Avenue South, New York, NY 10010-1710. Tel.: 212-633-3874; Fax: 212-633-3820; E-mail: reprints@elsevier.com.

Clinics in Podiatric Medicine and Surgery is covered in *MEDLINE/PubMed (Index Medicus)* and *EMBASE/Excerpta Medica*.

Contributors

CONSULTING EDITOR

THOMAS J. CHANG, DPM
Clinical Professor and Past Chairman, Department of Podiatric Surgery, California College of Podiatric Medicine, Faculty, The Podiatry Institute, Redwood Orthopedic Surgery Associates, Santa Rosa, California

EDITOR

MICHAEL H. THEODOULOU, DPM, FACFAS
Division Chief of Podiatric Surgery, Cambridge Health Alliance, Instructor of Surgery, Harvard Medical School, Somerville, Massachusetts

AUTHORS

LAURA B. ADLER, DPM
2nd Year Resident-Highlands-Presbyterian, St. Luke's Podiatric Medicine and Surgery Residency Program, Denver, Colorado

RACHEL H. ALBRIGHT, DPM, MPH, AACFAS
Attending Surgeon, Stamford Health Medical Group, Stamford, Connecticut

ANDREW M. BELIS, DPM, FACFAS, FASPS
Fellowship Director, Orthopedic Center of Florida, Fort Myers, Florida

ALAN J. BLOCK, DPM, MS, FACFAS
Williamsburg Foot Center, Kingstree, South Carolina

JENNIFER L. BUCHANAN, DPM, MS
Attending Podiatric Surgeon, Division of Podiatric Surgery, Cambridge Health Alliance, Massachusetts

MICHELLE L. BUTTERWORTH, DPM, FACFAS
Williamsburg Foot Center, Kingstree, South Carolina

ALAN CATANZARITI, DPM, FACFAS
Program Director, West Penn Hospital Foot and Ankle Surgery, Section Chief of Podiatry, Department of Orthopedic Surgery, Allegheny Health Network, Pittsburgh, Pennsylvania

ROBERT J. CAVALIERE, DPM
3rd Year Resident-Highlands-Presbyterian, St. Luke's Podiatric Medicine and Surgery Residency Program, Denver, Colorado

ADAM E. FLEISCHER, DPM, MPH, FACFAS
Director of Research, Weil Foot and Ankle Institute, Chicago, Illinois; Professor, Dr. William M. Scholl College of Podiatric Medicine, Rosalind Franklin University of Medicine and Science, North Chicago, Illinois

GREGORY A. FOOTE, DPM, AACFAS
Orthopedic Center of Florida, Fort Myers, Florida

DANIEL J. HATCH, DPM, FACFAS
Director of Surgery, North Colorado Podiatric Medical Surgical Residency, Greeley, Colorado

JACOB JONES, DPM
Resident Physician, Department of Orthopedics, Division of Foot and Ankle Surgery, West Penn Hospital, Foot and Ankle Institute, Pittsburgh, Pennsylvania

JASON KAYCE, DPM, FACFAS
Assistant Professor, Midwestern University Arizona College of Podiatric Medicine, Paradise Valley Foot & Ankle, Phoenix, Arizona

KARAN MALANI, DPM
Resident Physician, Cambridge Health Alliance, Cambridge, Massachusetts, USA

JOHN T. MARCOUX, DPM, DABFAS, FACFAS
Division of Podiatry, Department of Surgery, Beth Israel Deaconess Medical Center, Clinical Instructor in Surgery, Harvard Medical School, Boston, Massachusetts

SARA MATEEN, DPM
Resident, Temple University Hospital Podiatric Surgical Residency Program, Philadelphia, Pennsylvania

JEFFREY E. McALISTER, DPM, FACFAS
Attending, Phoenix Foot and Ankle Institute, Scottsdale, Arizona

ANDREW J. MEYR, DPM, FACFAS
Clinical Professor, Department of Podiatric Surgery, Temple University School of Podiatric Medicine, Philadelphia, Pennsylvania

KELLY M. PIROZZI, DPM, FACFAS
Chief, Podiatry, Director Podiatric Resident Training, Phoenix VA Healthcare System, Phoenix, Arizona

MADISON RAVINE, DPM
Resident Physician, Cambridge Health Alliance, Cambridge, Massachusetts, USA

DOUGLAS H. RICHIE Jr. DPM, FACFAS
Associate Clinical Professor, California School of Podiatric Medicine at Samuel Merritt University, Oakland, California

BRETT D. SACHS, DPM, FACFAS
Rocky Mountain Foot & Ankle Center, Wheat Ridge, Colorado; Program Director, Highlands-Presbyterian, St. Luke's Podiatric Medicine and Surgery Residency Program, Denver, Colorado

LAURA E. SANSOSTI, DPM, FACFAS
Clinical Associate Professor, Department of Podiatric Surgery, Temple University School of Podiatric Medicine, Philadelphia, Pennsylvania

HARRY P. SCHNEIDER, DPM
Residency Director and Attending Physician, Cambridge Health Alliance, Cambridge, Massachusetts, USA

LOWELL TONG, DPM, PMSR/RRA PGY-3
Division of Podiatry, Department of Surgery, Beth Israel Deaconess Medical Center, Boston, Massachusetts

Contents

> Fibrocartilage is a transitional tissue that derives from mesenchymal tissue that lacks a perichondrium and has structural and functional properties between that of dense fibrous connective tissue and hyaline cartilage. It is comprised of densely braided collagen fibers with a low number of chondrocytes that make the tissue highly resistant to compression. It contains high levels of Type I Collagen in addition to Type II Collagen and a small component of ground substance. It is dynamic in that its composition can change over time as it responds to local mechanical stresses and exposure to various cytologic chemicals. There are 4 main categories of fibrocartilage. The first is intra-articular whereby flexion and extension occur with gliding. The second is connecting fibrocartilage to disperse pressure across a joint. The third is stratiform which is a thin layer over a bone whereby tendon glides. The fourth is circumferential which is ring shaped. Various examples are discussed within this article.

> There are 3 types of cartilage found in the human body: hyaline cartilage, elastic cartilage, and fibrocartilage. Fibrocartilage may be found in intervertebral discs, symphysis pubis, tendinous insertions, acetabular labrums, and the temporomandibular joint. Specifically, in the foot and ankle we mainly see fibrocartilage in tendinous insertions and in areas where tendons wrap around boney prominence. Histologically, fibrocartilage is comprised of an extracellular matrix that contains glycosaminoglycans, proteoglycans, and collagens. This composition allows for a hydrophilic environment, which allows tissue to withstand high compressive forces seen in weight bearing.

> This article provides an update on fibrocartilaginous disease clinical examination. Lesser metatarsophalangeal joint instability is a challenging entity for the foot and ankle surgeon. A correct diagnosis is crucial to instill an appropriate treatment plan that will result in a successful outcome and a

satisfied patient. Insertional Achilles tendon disorders are common among active and inactive patients. There is also a high predilection for Achilles tendon pathology among athletes. In this article demographics and patient history, causative factors, differential diagnosis, physical examination, clinical tests, and radiographic evaluation are discussed for plantar plate disorders and insertional Achilles disorders.

This article provides an overview of the soft tissue contributions to the normal structures that surround the talo-calcaneal-navicular (TCN) joint of the human arch. The TCN joint has a multiplanar range of motion that makes it essential to the kinetic coupling that links the forefoot and hindfoot. The soft tissue connection surrounding this joint is known as the spring ligament complex. More accurate knowledge of the anatomy of this complex will enhance the understanding of its role in the support of the head of the talus and, potentially, its critical interactions with the normal or abnormal function of the arch.

The Achilles tendon is well known as the strongest tendon within the body. Its anatomic composition is unique to allow absorption of extreme loads. Historically, there has been a longstanding belief that rupture of the Achilles tendon occurs within a "watershed" region of ischemia. However, experimental data have demonstrated uniform hemodynamic flow throughout the tendon to challenge this widespread notion.

The fibrocartilaginous component of the plantar plate offers stability at the metatarsophalangeal joint. In conjunction with the attachments of the deep transverse metatarsal ligaments and collateral ligaments, the plantar plate complex resists tensile forces anchored by the plantar fascia and compression forces under the metatarsal heads.

The lesser metatarsophalangeal joint plantar plate and calcaneonavicular (spring) ligament are highly specialized soft tissue structures within the foot, consisting partly of fibrocartilage and capable of withstanding high compressive and tensile loads. Preoperative advanced imaging, in the form of point-of-care ultrasound and MRI, has become indispensable for surgeons hoping to confirm, quantify, and better localize injuries to these structures before surgery. This article describes the technical considerations of ultrasound and MRI and provides examples of the normal and abnormal appearances of these structures. The pros and cons of each imaging modality are also discussed.

Tendons and ligaments are critical components in the function of the musculoskeletal system, as they provide stability and guide motion for the biomechanical transmission of forces into bone. Several common injuries in the foot and ankle require the repair of ruptured or attenuated tendon or ligament to its osseous insertion. Understanding the structure and function of injured ligaments and tendons is complicated by the variability and unpredictable nature of their healing. The healing process at the tendon/ligament to bone interface is challenging and often frustrating to foot and ankle surgeons, as they have a high failure rate necessitating the need for revision.

The plantar plate is a critical structure involved in stabilizing the metatarsophalangeal joint. Its disruption can not only be painful for the patient but also may lead to subsequent structural deformities. There are several conservative treatment modalities available to help mitigate symptoms including splinting, offloading, and intraarticular injections. That being said, once the pathology progresses to advanced stages, these treatments are not efficacious. Reported success with conservative treatment modalities is limited to case studies and series with a low level of clinical evidence. As such, this represents an area where further investigation is needed to evaluate the true efficacy of conservative treatment and to allow for development of a more standardized approach.

The fibrocartilage within the superomedial calcaneonavicular (spring) ligament is part of an interwoven complex of ligaments that span the ankle, subtalar, and talonavicular joints. Acute isolated rupture of the spring ligament has been reported in association with an eversion ankle sprain. Attenuation and failure of the spring ligament causes complex 3D changes called the progressive collapsing foot deformity (PCFD). This deformity is characterized by hindfoot eversion, forefoot supination, collapse of the medial longitudinal arch, and forefoot abduction. Nonoperative treatment of an isolated spring ligament rupture and PCFD using various designs of orthoses have shown promising results.

Insertional Achilles tendinopathy can be a very challenging clinical syndrome with various nonoperative measures typically attempted before surgical intervention. Associated complications are known with surgical repair and can be limb altering. Owing to the longevity of clinical symptoms before clinical presentation, changing the pathophysiologic process and halting the inflammatory changes becomes paramount. Here we discuss nonoperative techniques and updates in the foot and ankle literature.

CLINICS IN PODIATRIC MEDICINE AND SURGERY

SERIES OF RELATED INTEREST

Orthopedic Clinics
https://www.orthopedic.theclinics.com/
Clinics in Sports Medicine
https://www.sportsmed.theclinics.com/
Foot and Ankle Clinics
https://www.foot.theclinics.com/
Physical Medicine and Rehabilitation Clinics
https://www.pmr.theclinics.com/

THE CLINICS ARE AVAILABLE ONLINE!
Access your subscription at:
www.theclinics.com

Foreword

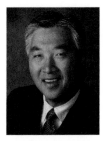

Thomas J. Chang, DPM
Consulting Editor

It is my pleasure to introduce this issue on fibrocartilaginous disease. As foot and ankle surgeons, we fully appreciate the contributions of soft tissue to almost every structural and positional deformity we encounter. We know what appears to be a "simple" bunion deformity is a 4-dimensional deformity with transverse, sagittal, frontal plane, and length concerns. This is a combination of a bone and soft tissue pathologic condition, and both need to be considered. There are often biomechanical stresses imparted to the lesser metatarsal phalangeal joints and flexor/plantar plate injuries are common.

Is there a "simple" flatfoot deformity? The flatfoot is a complex combination of osseous and soft tissue changes, and we are intimately aware of how important the spring ligament is and the vital role it plays in the early to later stages of the deformity. It is also well understood the Achilles tendon plays a vital role in the majority of foot and ankle pathologic conditions. We commonly address the Achilles with forefoot, midfoot, and hindfoot deformities.

This issue focuses on truly understanding the complexity of these fibrocartilaginous soft tissues and their disease states. The ultimate goal is to enhance our awareness of how this tissue behaves in each anatomic location, the nuances that might improve healing, and considerations to improve long-term outcomes in each situation.

I know Dr Theodoulou has been passionate about this topic for many years. He is a critical thinker and has tremendous resources around him at Harvard Medical School. I am excited to see his journey into this specialized area of fibrocartilaginous diseases and his desire to share his work with us. I know our patients will be better for it. Enjoy this issue.

Thomas J. Chang, DPM
Redwood Orthopedic Surgery Associates
208 Concourse Boulevard
Santa Rosa, CA 95403, USA

E-mail address:
thomaschang14@comcast.net

Clin Podiatr Med Surg 39 (2022) xi
https://doi.org/10.1016/j.cpm.2022.04.001
0891-8422/22/© 2022 Published by Elsevier Inc.

Preface

Update on Fibrocartilaginous Disease

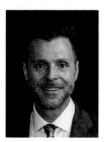

Michael H. Theodoulou, DPM, FACFAS
Editor

It is an honor to serve as a guest editor for *Clinics in Podiatric Medicine and Surgery* and to present on a topic that impacts with regularity lower extremity physicians and their patients. Fibrocartilage disorders are the cause of several derangements identified the human foot. I have had great interest in this topic. The ability to restore the normal physiologic function of this tissue without other sacrifices makes it an ongoing challenge. The development of lesser metatarsophalangeal joint instability and progression of the digital deformity, advancing collapse of the foot resulting from spring ligament failure, and chronic pain to the posterior aspect of the heel result from the unique characteristics of this tissue. In this text, we review the gross and histologic anatomy of the plantar plate, the spring ligament, and the Achilles tendon. We appreciate their anatomy and influence on the physiology and mechanics of this tissue. The authors identify clinical assessment of the tissue in disease. We consider the presentation on imaging to assist in diagnosis, prognosis, and recommended management. Treatment options, nonoperative and operative, are outlined. Finally, we appreciate when and why there is a failure in our care and how we can manage it. I have been fortunate to have assembled an incredible group of contributors to assist in this

Clin Podiatr Med Surg 39 (2022) xiii–xiv
https://doi.org/10.1016/j.cpm.2022.03.005
0891-8422/22/© 2022 Published by Elsevier Inc.

endeavor. Through their experience and research, we will try to provide better insight into the care of this tissue.

Michael H. Theodoulou, DPM, FACFAS
Cambridge Health Alliance
Harvard Medical School
1493 Cambridge Street
Cambridge, MA 02139, USA

E-mail address:
mtheodoulou@challiance.org

Types of Fibrocartilage

Jennifer L. Buchanan, DPM, MS

KEYWORDS

- Fibrochondrocytes • Mesenchymal stem cells • Chondrogenesis • Metaplasia

KEY POINTS

- Chondrogenesis is a dynamic process involving mesenchymal stem cell recruitment, migration, condensation of progenitor cells, chondrocyte differentiation, proliferation, hypertrophy, and angiogenesis.
- Types of fibrocartilage: Intra-articular, connecting, stratiform, circumferential.
- Function: Reduction of compression forces and strain in areas with high levels of wear and tear.

INTRODUCTION

Fibrocartilage is a transitional tissue that lacks a perichondrium and has structural and functional properties between that of dense fibrous connective tissue and hyaline cartilage. It serves as a tough dense material and is comprised of densely braided collagen fibers with a low number of chondrocytes that make the tissue highly resistant to compression.[1,2] It contains high levels of Type I Collagen in addition to Type II Collagen and a small component of ground substance. This varies from hyaline cartilage which is primarily comprised of Type II Collagen thus resulting in different functions in the body. Depending on its location, fibrocartilage is comprised of varying levels of collagen and fibrous tissue.[3] It is also dynamic in that its composition can change over time as it responds to local mechanical stresses and exposure to various cytologic chemicals. The embryologic development, location, and types of fibrocartilage and their general function currently known will be discussed in this section.

EMBRYOLOGIC DEVELOPMENT

Cartilage is a mesenchymal derivative that begins to form during the fifth gestational week. Joint development is marked by the appearance of a region of flattened, condensed cells at putative joint sites called the interzone. This has 3 layers including an intermediate zone consisting of dense, flattened cells in between layers of chondrogenic cells. Joint cavitation occurs in the center of the interzone and the cells and their surroundings gradually form articular cartilage.[4]

Division of Podiatric Surgery, Cambridge Health Alliance, 1493 Cambridge Street, Cambridge, MA 02139, USA
E-mail address: jlbuchanan@challiance.org

Clin Podiatr Med Surg 39 (2022) 357–361
https://doi.org/10.1016/j.cpm.2022.02.001
0891-8422/22/© 2022 Elsevier Inc. All rights reserved.

There are 2 primary ways that fibrocartilage develops: either through differentiation from immature hyaline cartilage or differentiation from dense fibrous connective tissue. As such, it is difficult to classify the cells from which it is comprised. Sometimes they are referred to as fibrocartilage cells, fibrochondrocytes, or fibroblasts.

Adult human bone marrow-derived mesenchymal stromal cells (hMSCs) are at default committed toward osteogenesis. Chondrogenesis, which comprises cartilage development, involves several regulated events as depicted in **Fig. 1**. First, the mesenchymal stem cells (MSCs) are committed to become cartilage cells. They produce extracellular matrix (ECM) containing hyaluronan and collagens I, II, III, V, IX, and XI.[5,6] The MSCs undergo "condensation" to a more compact nodule called a chondrocyte.[7] Packing of the cells tight together initiates gap-junction mediated cell–cell communication which initiates chondrogenesis and differentiation of the surrounding MSCs into chondrocytes.[8] Important factors involved in the process of differentiation include cell transcription factors such as Smads, p38, RhoA/ROCK, and SOX9.[9] Additionally, 2 important cell adhesion molecules in this process are neural cadherin and neural cell adhesion molecule (N-CAM).[10] Chondrocytes are then stimulated to proliferate rapidly and produce more ECM. Chondrocytes then undergo hypertrophy and begin to express collagen Type X and alkaline phosphatase.[11] In areas of bone development, the chondrocytes are infiltrated by vascular penetration and replaced by osteoblasts to form bone. At the end of long bones, the chondrocytes proliferate before undergoing hypertrophy pushing out the cartilaginous ends of the bone whereby cartilage remains relatively inactive largely due to poor vascularity and innervation.[12] Signals such as bone morphogenic protein (BMP), Indian hedgehog (Ihh), and parathyroid hormone-related peptide (PTHrP) are involved in pushing these embryonic progenitors toward articular cartilage formation instead of ossification. Other ECM molecules additionally regulate chondrogenesis. For example, selective inhibition of BMP receptors has been shown to result in MSC differentiation to chondrocytes.[13] Fibronectin is increased in areas of cellular condensation and then is reduced as cell differentiation occurs thus also playing a role in the differentiation to chondrocyte production.[14] There has been a great deal of research on factors that promote chondrogenesis given the significant morbidity associated with osteoarthritis but challenges remain in targeting this physiologic phenomenon. ECM production switches rapidly from collagen type I to type IIa and there is an increase in the production of sulfated proteoglycans including aggrecan, which constitute most of the environment surrounding mature chondrocytes in cartilage.These function to retain water and maintain distance between cells and serve as shock absorbers.[15]

Fibrocartilage can subsequently develop from these immature hyaline cartilage cells. They are similar to chondrocytes in that they possess a round to oval shape

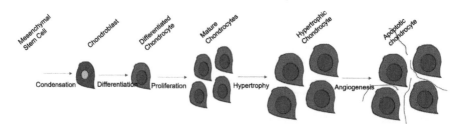

Fig. 1. Chondrogenesis begins from the condensation of MSCs into chondroblast which undergoes differentiation to Differentiated Chondrocyte, then proliferation to become mature chondrocyte which then hypertrophies and further undergoes angiogenesis.

and are isolated within lacunae in the ECM but they lack the gap junctions and therefore have no communication between them. When fibrocartilage develops from mesenchymal tissue, an increased fibrous content precedes the appearance of cartilage cells.[16] The cells possess lipid droplets, glycogen granules, and multiple intermediate filaments which help the cells tolerate compressive forces. This makes fibrocartilage a more appropriate structure in areas of compressive loading such as in the spine or in the mensci.[17] Fibrocartilage may also develop later by metaplasia of precartilage, hyaline cartilage, and fibrous tissue. It can be arranged in different patterns depending on location but tends to derive from young cells in the area of strain. The knee menisci contain circumferential hoops. In the regions of tendons that base around bone pulleys, the collagen fibers have a basket-weave appearance and some bundles run at right angles to the long axis of the tendon.[1]

TYPES OF FIBROCARTILAGE

There are 4 main categories of fibrocartilage which will be discussed here and a review of the locations whereby they may be found within the human body is also discussed. The first category is intra-articular cartilage which is located at joints whereby flexion and extension are associated with gliding. They help to prevent joint instability. An example of this would be the menisci. The second category is connecting fibrocartilage which is located at limited motion joints, acting as a cushion to distribute stress across the joint. An example would be the intervertebral discs. The third form is

Table 1	
Location and function of fibrocartilage in the human body	
Location	**Function**
Secondary cartilaginous joints • Public Symphysis • Annulus fibrosis of intervertebral discs, tympanic membrane • Manubriosternal joint • TMJ-develop fibrocartilaginous articular surface at approximately 17-20 years[1]	
Glenoid labrum shoulder joint	
Acetabular labrum joint	The fibrocartilage lip deepens the acetabular ring and distributes forces by maintaining synovial fluid between the articular surfaces. Also prevents lateral translation of the femoral head.
Medical and lateral menisci of the knee	Prevention of joint stability
Tendon/ligament attachments to bone • Superior portion of the posterior calcaneus where the Achilles tendon inserts • Posterior tibial tendon at its insertion on the navicula	Reduces stress from the enthesis to reduce wear and tear[2]
Plantar plate of fingers and toes[18] Spring ligament of the foot[20]	Disperse strain in areas of high flexion
Ligamentum arteriosum and central fibrous body of the heart, aortic and pulmonary valves[19]	

stratiform fibrocartilage. The is comprised of a thin layer of fibrocartilage over a bone whereby a tendon glides to help reduce fraction. For example, underlying the peroneal longus tendon whereby it glides across the bones. Lastly, there is circumferential fibrocartilage. This is a ring-shaped area of fibrous cartilage which protects the joint margins and improves bony fit such as in the acetabular labrum.[21]

LOCATION AND FUNCTION

Fibrocartilage is located throughout the body, especially in regions of enthesis or wrap-around regions (whereby tendons or ligaments make bends). **Table 1** lists in detail locations that are reported throughout the literature. The mechanical properties are intermediate between hyaline and elastic cartilage. The tensile strength of fibrocartilage is roughly 10 MPa which is less than that of a tendon but great than hyaline cartilage.[22]

Fibrocartilage is also involved in the healing of articular cartilage and bone or tendon. If defects in the avascular region of the meniscus are filled with an exogenous fibrin clot, the wound is healed and fibrous tissue appears which undergoes metaplasia to fibrocartilage.[23] The fibrocartilage arises from cancellous bone or synovial pannus but is not derived from articular cartilage at the edges of the defect.[24] The fibrocartilage in wrap-around tendons is located within the fascicles, epitenon, or endotenon.[2] It is debated whether its presence is a result of wear and tear and pathologic development or whether its presence is just a normal result of compression and strain.[16] Tendons that wrap around the ankle are distinctly fibrocartilaginous as they are constantly bent around bone and act like pulleys that are under heavier loads.[16] Tendons that attach to the epiphysis of long bones or to the short bones of the tarsus have fibrocartilaginous enthesis as well, again potentially as a protective mechanism of these areas.

CLINICS CARE POINTS

- Fibrocartilage is located in many places throughout the body that have high levels of stress and strain.
- Knowing the locations of these types of fibrocartilage may allow us to target specific treatment modalities in the future.

DISCLOSURE

The author has nothing to disclose.

REFERENCES

1. Benjamin M, Evans EJ. Fibrocartilage. J Anat 1990;171:1–15.
2. Benjamin M, Ralphs JR. Biology of fibrocartilage cells. Int Rev Cytol 2004; 223:1–45.
3. Armiento AR, Alini M, Stoddart MJ. Articular cartilage- why does hyaline cartilage fail to repair? Adv Drug Deliv Rev 2019;146:289–305.
4. Mitrovic DR. Development of the metatarsophalangeal joint of the chick embryo: morphological, ultrastructural and histochemical studies. Am J Anat 1977;150(2): 333–47.

5. Goldring MB. Chondrogenesis, chondrocyte differentiation, and articular carti- lage metabolism in health and osteoarthritis. Ther Adv Musculoskeleta Dis 2012;4(4):269–85.
6. Hall BK, Miyake T. The membranous skeleton: the role of cell condensations in vertebrate skeletogenesis. Anat Embryol 1992;186:107–24.
7. Gruneberg H. The pathology of development: a study of inherited skeletal disor- ders in animal. Oxford (United Kingdom): Blackwarells Scientifc publications; 1963.
8. San Antonio JD, Tuan RS. Chrondrogenesis of limb bud mesenchyme in vitro: stimulation by cations. Dev lol 1986;115:313–24.
9. Griffin M, Hindocha S, Khan WS. Chondrogenic differentiation of adult MSCs. Curr Stem Cell Res Ther 2012;7(4):260–5.
10. Oberlander S, Tuan RS. Expression and functional involvement of N-cadherin in embryonic limb chondrogenesis. Development 1994;120:177–87.
11. Johnstone B, Hering TM, Caplan AI, et al. In Vitro Chrondogenesis of bone marrow-derived mesenchymal progenitor cells. Exp Cell Res 1998;238(1): 265–72.
12. Chen Q, Johnson DM, Haudenschild DR, et al. Progression and recapitulation of the chondrocyte differentiation program: cartilage matrix protein is a marker for cartilage maturation. Dev Biol 1995;172:293–306.
13. Ochetta P, Pigeot S, Rasponi M, et al. Developmentally inspired programming of adult human mesenchymal stromal cells toward stable chondrogenesis. Proc Natl Acad Sci U S A 2018;115:4625–30.
14. Kulyk WM, Upholt WB, Kosher RA. Fibronectin gene expression during limb carti- lage differentiation. Development 1989;106:449–55.
15. Solursh M, Ahrens PB, Retier RS. A tissue culture analysis of the steps in limb chondrogenesis. In Vitro 1978;14:51–61.
16. Benjamin M, Ralphs JR. Fibrocartilage in tendons and ligaments- an adaptation to compressive load. J Anat 1998;193:481–94.
17. Wren TAL, Beaupre GS, Carter DR. Mechanobiology of tendon adaptation to compressive loading through fibrocartilaginous metaplasia. J Rhab Res Develop 2000;37(2):135–44.
18. Norregaard O, Jakobsen J, Nielsen KK. Hyperextension injuries of the PIP finger joint. Comparison of early motion and immobilization. Acta orthopaedics Scand 1987;58:239–40.
19. Balogh K. Fibrocartilage in the heart. Lancet 1971;i:802.
20. Hodges Davis W, Sobel M, DiCarlo EF. Gross, Histological, and microvascular anatomy and biomechanical testing of the spring ligament complex. Foot Ankle Int 1996;17(2):95–102.
21. Crumbie L. Fibrocartilage. Available at: https://www.kenhub.com/en/library/ anatomy/fibrocartilage. Accessed August 8, 2021.
22. Yamada H. Strength of biological materials. Baltimore (MD): Williams & Wilkins; 1970.
23. Arnoczky SP, Adams ME, DeHaven KE, Eyre DR, Mow VC. The meniscus. In: Woo SL-Y, Buckwalter J, editors. Injury and Repair of Musculoskeletal Soft Tis- sues. Park Ridge, IL: American Academy of Orthopaedic Surgeons; 1987. p. 487–537.
24. Meachum G, Roberts C. Repair of the joint surface from subarticular tissue in the rabbit knee. J Anat 1971;109:317–27.

Histophysiology of Fibrocartilage

Kelly M. Pirozzi, DPM, FACFAS

KEYWORDS

• Cartilage • Collagen • Disc • Fibrocartilage • Glycoaminoglycans

KEY POINTS

- Fibrocartilage can be found in intervertebral discs, symphysis pubis, menisci, tendinous insertions, the glenohumeral/acetabular labrum, and the temporomandibular joint.
- Fibrocartilage is reinforced with parallel bundles of collagen fibers, which in turn make it the strongest type of cartilage.
- The composition of the extracellular matrix allows for high water content, which allows fibrocartilage to withstand high compressive forces.

INTRODUCTION

The fundamental knowledge of treating fibrocartilaginous disease lies first with the understanding of the complex fibrocartilage histophysiology. By understanding the basic science behind fibrocartilage and more generally cartilage, we are better able to treat and manage musculoskeletal injuries and pathology. Fibrocartilage aids in joint stability and the body's ability to withstand high compressive forces. It consists of many diverse functions throughout the body and can be found in tissue such as menisci, intervertebral discs, ligaments, tendons, and joints such as the temporal mandibular joint.[1] We are particularly interested in fibrocartilage in foot and ankle surgery, as tendons and ligaments play an integral role in biomechanics and stability. Where tendon and ligaments are subject to compression, they are frequently attached to boney regions with fibrocartilaginous tissue.[2] When this system breaks down, it can lead to instability and pathology within the foot and ankle. Our ability to restore function in these regions should first rely on a basic understanding of the histophysiology of these tissues.

The fibrocartilage within tendons and ligaments can be located within fascicles or in endo/epitenon.[2] They are commonly packed with intermediate filaments that assist in mechanical loading. Intermediate filaments may be able to resist high mechanical load through interactions between the cytoskeleton, integrins within the cell membranes, and the extracellular matrix.[2,3] Fibrocartilage that is present in the epitenon or

Phoenix VA Healthcare System, 650 E Indian School Road, Phoenix, AZ 85012, USA
E-mail address: kellypirozzi@gmail.com

Clin Podiatr Med Surg 39 (2022) 363–370
https://doi.org/10.1016/j.cpm.2022.02.002
0891-8422/22/Published by Elsevier Inc.

endotenon may protect the tendons' vasculature by allowing fascicles to slide over each other in malleable areas of the tendon, where fibrocartilage located within the fascicle may be surrounded by an interwoven network of collagen.[2] Enthesis fibrocartilage is found at the point where tendons and ligaments attach to bone. Fibrocartilage is also noted in areas where the tendon changes direction by wrapping around boney pulleys. The extracellular matrix in these areas has high levels of aggrecan and type II collagen, which allow for high compression forces.[2]

On a molecular level, the histophysiology of fibrocartilage is a complex, intricate system that plays an integral role synthesizing a variety of matrix molecules including collagens, proteoglycans, and noncollagenous proteins.[1] By obtaining better knowledge of the histophysiology and role each of the molecules play, we can better understand their function in the body. Using this understanding, advances in science may be made in order to replicate this system in order to address pathologies in the foot and ankle.

WHAT IS CARTILAGE?

Cartilage plays an integral part of the musculoskeletal system in order to reinforce weight-bearing joints. Cartilage is avascular and aneural, which allows it to provide dense support that can withstand compressive forces. Unlike bone, it is still able to bend and have some flexibility and remain malleable, which makes it ideal for joints and areas of high stress. Although being avascular and aneural may have many benefits with regard to shock absorption and weight-bearing, it may also plague us when this system fails and needs to be repaired. Trying to restore the normal histophysiology of fibrocartilage is challenging, and advances in biologics continue to attempt to replicate the body's natural regeneration process.

Cartilage is made up of a composition of chondroblasts, chondrocytes, fibrochondrocytes, and extracellular matrix (ECM). The composition of which of these molecules and what quantity exists depends on the function and type of cartilage; however, it is the ECM that makes up most of the cartilage in general. On a very basic level, the ECM is made up of gylcosaminoglycans (GAGs) that are linked together by proteins (proteoglycans).[4] The composition of the ECM (which may include elastic fibers, collagen, proteoglycans, and GAGs) can differ slightly between tissue types, and this is what gives each subtype of cartilage its unique biomechanical properties. Overall, the ECM is very good at absorbing water through osmosis, which leads to its high water content. This high water content is what allows the ECM and thus cartilage to resist compressive forces. Each of these components found in cartilage is investigated further.

- *Chondroblasts:* chondroblasts are *immature* cells that aid in cartilage development. They may also be known as perichondrial cells or mesenchymal progenitor cells, which give rise to chondrocytes.
- *Chondrocytes:* chondrocytes are *mature* cells typically found in the matrix cavities called lacunae. Their main function is to produce, maintain, and remodel the cartilage; this process is called chondrogenesis. They are able to adjust and remodel by sensing and responding to changes in mechanical loads.[5] Chondrocytes are embedded within the ECM and contain ion channels that aid in mechanotransduction mediated through PIEZO1 and TRPV4.[5] These cells can sense changes in mechanical loading and respond by adjusting with anabolic or catabolic processes in order to maintain structure of the cartilage tissue.[5] It is important to preserve balance between the anabolic and catabolic processes to maintain normal tissue physiology.

- *Fibrochondrocytes:* fibrochondrocytes are cells that produce fibrocartilage. They may resemble chondrocytes in that they are isolated within the lacunae of the extracellular matrix. Fibrochondrocytes consist of lipid droplets, glycogen granules, and intermediate filaments. These intermediate filaments help to reinforce the components of the fibrochondrocytes that allow the surrounding tissue to tolerate greater compressive forces.[5]
- *GAGs:* GAGs are unbranched polysaccharide chains. These chains are made up of long repeating disaccharide units, one of which is always an amino sugar (hence glyco*AMINO*glycan). GAGs are highly negatively charged, which aids in osmosis and makes them strongly hydrophilic by drawing water into the ECM. Unlike proteins, they are long chains that are inflexible.[4]
  - *Hyaluronan (hyaluronic acid, hyaluronate):* this is the simplest *nonsulfated* GAG and longest chain. Because it is so large, it absorbs water and swells up a large area or volume, which makes it a good space filler as well as a good shock absorber for weight-bearing.

The following 3 GAGs are small and *complex sulfated sugars*.

  - *Chondroitin sulfate/dermatan sulfate*: chondroitin sulfate and dermatan sulfate consist of the repeating disaccharide *N-acetylglucosamine* and hexuronic acids (iduronic acid vs glucuronic acid).[6] Chondroitin sulfate contains a rubbery consistency, which provides cartilage with its resilience.
  - *Heparan sulfate/heparin*: heparin sulfate and heparin contain repeating disaccharide units of *N-acetylgalactosamine* and hexuronic acids (glucuronic acid vs iduronic acid).[6]
  - *Keratan sulfate*: keratan sulfate contains the repeating disaccharide of galactose and *N-acetylglucosamine.* Keratan sulfate is the only sulfated GAG that is not connected to the proteoglycan protein core by a tetrasaccharide linker compound.[6]
- *Proteoglycans:* proteoglycans are GAGs that are attached to a core protein (except hyaluronic acid). Proteoglycans have a negative charge, therefore attracting positively charged ions, specifically sodium (Na+). Through this osmotic process, water is transferred into the ECM. Proteoglycans may also aid in storing growth factors and aid in regulation of enzymes. When specifically looking at the role of proteoclycans in fibrocartilage, they are relatively scarce, which makes the tissue seem relatively more acidophilic when compared with hyaline or elastic extracellular matrix composition. Overall, proteoglycans make up approximately 1% of the tensile weight of tendons.[7] The proteoglycans found in tendons are classified into 2 groups:
  - *Small leucine-rich proteoglycans (SLRPs)*: the main proteoglycan present in tendon is decorin. Decorin makes up 80% of total proteoglycan content in tendons. Other SLRPs may include biglycan, fibromodulin, lumican, and keratocan.[7]
  - *Large aggregating proteoglycans*: the large aggregating proteoglycans found in the tensional region of tendons include aggrecan and versican[7]; these characteristically contain globular domains separated by a GAG attachment region.[7]

There are 3 different types of cartilage: hyaline cartilage, fibrocartilage, and elastic cartilage. These 3 types of cartilage share basic molecular components; however, they vary in composition and utility (**Table 1**).

- *Hyaline cartilage:* hyaline cartilage is the most common type of cartilage. It contains a glassy appearance.
- *Elastic cartilage:* elastic cartilage contains elastic fibers as well as collagen fibers, which give it its characteristic functions of flexibility and resilience.

Table 1
Three different types of cartilage

	Hyaline Cartilage	Elastic Cartilage	Fibrocartilage
Extracellular Matrix (ECM)	• Type II collagen • Aggrecan • Chondrocytes • Chondroblasts • Small isogenous groups	• Type II collagen • Aggrecan • Chondrocytes • Chondroblasts • Dark elastic Fibers • Small isogenous groups	• Type 1 & II collagen • Dense connective tissue • Fibrochondrocytes • Axially arranged isogenous groups
Locations	• Epiphyseal plates and articular ends of long bones • Fetal skeleton • Upper respiratory tract	• External ear • Auditory tube • Epiglottis • Laryngeal cartilage	• Intervertebral discs • Symphysis pubis • Menisci • Tendinous insertions • Glenohumeral/acetabular labrum • Temporomandibular joint
Functions	• Joint articulation • Scaffold for osteogenesis	• Structural support	• Weight-bearing • Compression/shear force resistance

- *Fibrocartilage:* this cartilage is responsible for tendinous insertions and intervertebral discs. It is reinforced with parallel bundles of collagen fibers, which in turn make it the strongest type. It also has alternating layers of hyaline cartilage matrix and thick layers of dense collagen fibers that are oriented in the direction of functional stresses. This composition allows for increased strength. Usually, fibrocartilage is a transitional layer between the hyaline cartilage and tendon/ligament.[4] An example of fibrocartilage clusters within tendon is demonstrated in **Fig. 1**.

HISTOLOGY OF FIBROCARTILAGE

Fibrocartilage is a dense orderly arrangement of cartilage fibers. Chondrocytes are located within the lacunae, spaces located between the ECM, and are spaced between the fibers. Fibrocartilage may be differentiated from dense connective tissue through the chondrocytes that are surrounded by the matrix.

Fibrocartilage is categorized into 4 different types:[4]

- Intaarticular fibrocartilage: an example of intraarticular fibrocartilage would be the menisci; these are present in joints that function with flexion and extension and aid in the gliding motion while acting padding to strengthen stability of the joint.
- Connecting fibrocartilage: an example of connecting fibrocartilage would be intervertebral discs. This type of cartilage is typically found in limited motion joints and typically act as a cushion to distribute stress more evenly.
- Stratiform fibrocartilage: stratiform fibrocartilage presents as a thin layer over bones, allowing tendons to glide around the bone more easily. An example of this would be minimizing friction between the peroneus longus and tibialis posterior as they course through the ankle and foot (**Fig. 2**).
- Circumferential fibrocartilage: circumferential fibrocartilage present as a ring around joint margins in order to provide a more secure bony fit at the joint. Examples of this would be the glenoid joint and the acetabular labrum.

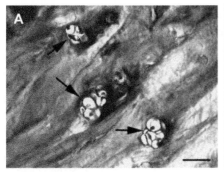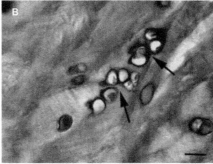

Fig. 1. (*A*) Arrows directed toward clusters of fibrocartilage cells from human Achilles tendon. (*B*) Arrows directed toward clusters of fibrocartilage cells from human Biceps brachii tendon. (*From* Benjamin M, Ralphs JR. Biology of fibrocartilage cells. Int Rev Cytol. 2004;233:1-45. https://doi.org/10.1016/S0074-7696(04)33001-9. PMID: 15037361.)

Collagen contributes up to almost half of the composition of cartilage. The most common cartilages found in the body are types I and II.[8] Quantity, size, and type of collagen fibers vary depending on the subtype of cartilage. For example, normal Achilles tendon consists of 95% type I collagen. The covalent bonds between the collagen molecules gives the tendon its high tensile strength.[9,10] Ruptured or injured tendons show a decrease in type I collagen and an increase in type III collagen.[9,11] Type III collagen demonstrates less tensile strength than type I collagen, which may predispose the tendon to injury or rupture.[12]

In normal tendon, proteoglycans in the ECM are often associated with collagen fibrils or hyaluronan. In addition, there are also noncollagenous proteins present in the ECM of tendons, which include elastin, link protein, cartilage oligomeric matrix protein, tenascin-C, fibronectin, and thrombospondin.[7] These noncollagenous proteins are responsible for matrix-matrix, cell-matrix organization, and signaling.

It is the tenocytes that are responsible for metabolism of the proteoglycans. With increased mechanical stress, tenocytes increase expression of proteoglycans and ECM molecules. There is a balance between synthesis and catabolism of these proteoglycans. Catabolism of proteoglycans within the tendon is mediated by aggrecanases where they can cleave aggrecan at certain sites.[7] The ECM of tendon fibrocartilage contains small-diameter collagen fibers and frequently type II collagen.[3]

Indirect tendons that wrap around boney areas have a much higher GAG content when compared with direct tendons.[3] This high GAG content is likely associated

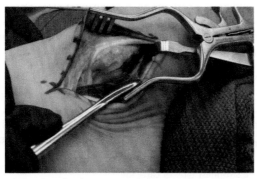

Fig. 2. The posterior lateral malleolar peroneal groove where the peroneal tendon wraps around the distal fibula.

with aggrecan, which is creating high osmotic pressure and increased water content to allow for increased compressive forces.

TENDINOPATHY

The structure of the ECM of tendon allows for the transmission of force generated by a muscle onto bone.[7] In pathologic tendons, the ECM is compromised, resulting in swelling and pain.[7] These tendons exhibit similar pathologic characteristics, which include increased levels of proteoglycans, water content, and collagen disorganization.[13–18] They have also been shown to have increased levels of SLRPs fibromodulin and biglycan.[7] These changes in SLRPs may contribute to degradation of the collagen network. There is also increased synthesis of large proteoglycans aggrecan and versican seen in tendinopathic tissue.[7,15,19]

Not only do we see variations of the collagen with injured versus healthy tendon but also there are noted differences seen with tendons with age. There is also a noted decrease in type I collagen during the normal aging process, which places our tendons at greater risk of rupture with age. In addition to changes in collagen, there is a change in fiber density and diameter with age that may also contribute to weakening of tensile strength and predispose the tendon to rupture and injury.[8,17]

Some studies have investigated specific collagen patterns that are at risk for tendinopathy. The crimp angle, which is the angular measure of the sinusoidal pattern of collagen in the tendon, has been correlated to tendons' ability to withstand sudden forces. The crimps in tendon fibers allow for a buffer within the tendon to avoid rupture from sudden stretch. Not only was there an observed decrease in crimp angle in ruptured tendons when compared with healthy tendons but there was also an observed decrease in crimp angle naturally with age.[20,24]

SUMMARY

Fibrocartilage has a relatively low quantity of type II and an abundance of type 1 collagen, which gives it its unique histologic feature. However, nonfibrillar collagen (types IX and XII) have also been documented in some fibrocartilages.[21] Nonfibrillar collagens influence the shape and fiber thickness of type 1 collagen, or they may aid in anchoring groups of fibers together and with surrounding tissues.[21–24]

On a molecular level, the ECM, fibrochondrocytes, chondrocytes, and chondroblasts work together to create an environment with high water content, which allows for the mechanical properties that fibrocartilage exhibits and allows for weight-bearing with greater compressive/shear force resistance. In the foot and ankle, we see fibrocartilage mainly in tendinous insertions as in areas where tendons wrap around boney prominences. When the balance of anabolic and catabolic processes fails, then the entire unit becomes pathologic. Better understanding of the histophysiology of normal fibrocartilage allows for better treatment in pathologic tissue.

CLINICS CARE POINTS

- Fibrocartilage can withstand high compressive forces.
- Fibrocartilage can be found at tendinous insertions and around boney prominences in the foot and ankle.
- Fibrocartilage is the strongest type of cartilage.

REFERENCES

1. Benjamin M, Ralphs JR. Biology of fibrocartilage cells. Int Rev Cytol 2004; 233:1–45.
2. Benjamin M, Ralphs JR. Fibrocartilage in tendons and ligaments- an adaptation to compressive load. J Anat 1998;193 481–494.
3. Benjamin M, Ralphs JR. Cytoskeleton of cartilage cells. Mircros Res Tech 1994; 28(5):372–7.
4. Peckham M, Knibbs A, Paxton S. The histology Guide: cartilage, Bone & Ossification. 2004. Hosted by the Facility of biological sciences at Leeds. Available at: https://www.histology.leeds.ac.uk/bone/cartilage.php. Accessed August 20, 2021.
5. Servin-Vences MR, Richardson J, Lewin GR, et al. Mechanoelectrical transduction in chondrocytes. Clin Exp Pharmacol Physiol 2018;45(5):481–8.
6. Casale J, Crane JS. Biochemistry, glycosaminoglycans. In: StatPearls [Internet]. Treasure Island (FL): StatPearls Publishing; 2021.
7. Parkinson J, Samiric T, Ilic MZ, et al. Involvement of proteoglycans in tendinopathy. J Musculoskelet Neuronal Interact 2011;11(2):86–93.
8. Wu F, Nerlick Michael, Denitsa Docheva. Tendon injuries; basic science and New repair Proposals. EFFORT Open Rev 2017;2(7):332–42.
9. Dederer KM, Tennant JN. Anatomical and functional Considerations in achilles tendon Lesions. Foot Ankle Clin 2019;24(3):371–85.
10. O'Brien M. Functional anatomy and physiology of tendons. Clin Sports Med 1992; 11(3):505–20.
11. Maffulli N. Tenocytes from ruptured and tendinopathic achilles tendons produce greater quantities of type III collagen than tenocytes from normal achilles tendons. An in vitro model of human tendon healing. Am J Sports Med 2000;28(4):499–505.
12. Waggett AD, Ralphs JR, Kwan AP, et al. Characterization of collagens and proteoglycans at the insertion of the human Achilles tendon. Matrix Biol 1998;16: 457–70.
13. Kannus P. Structure of the tendon connective tissue. Scand J Med Sci Sport 2000;(10):312–20.
14. de Mos M, van El B, DeGroot J, et al. Achilles tendinosis: changes in biochemical composition and collagen turnover rate. Am J Sports Med 2007;35:1549–56.
15. Scott A, Lian O, Roberts CR, et al. Increased versican content is associated with tendinosis pathology in the patellar tendon of athletes with jumper's knee. Scand J Med Sci Sports 2008;18:427–35.
16. Samiric T, Parkinson J, Ilic MZ, et al. Changes in the composition of the extracellular matrix in patellar tendinopathy. Matrix Biol 2009;28:230–6.
17. Pierre-Jerome C, Moncayo V, Terk MR. MRI of the Achilles tenon: a comprehensive review of the anatomy, biomechanics, and imaging of overuse tendinopathies. Acta Radiol 2010;51(4):438–54.
18. Winnicki K, Ochala-Klos A, Rutowicz B, et al. Functional anatomy, histology and biomechanics of the human Achilles tendon- A comprehensive review. Ann Anat 2020;229:151461.
19. Jarvinen TAH. Collagen fibres of the spontaneously ruptured human tendons display decreased thickness and crimp anlge. J Orthop Res 2004;22(6):1303–9.
20. Wong M. Kiel J. Anatomy, Lower limb, calf, tendons, Achilles. Treasure Island (FL): StatPearls; 2018.
21. Crumble L. Fibrocartilage. Last reviewed 2021. 2021. Available at: https://www. kenhub.com/en/library/anatomy/fibrocartilage. Accessed August 20th 2021.

22. Sophia Fox AJ, Bedi A, Rodeo SA. The basic science of articular cartilage: structure, composition, and function. Sports Health 2009;1(6):461–8.

23. Poole AR. What type of cartilage repair are we attempting to attain? J Bone Joint Surg Am 2003;85-A(Suppl 2):40–4.

24. Gaut L, Duprez D. Tendon development and diseases. Wiley Interdiscip Rev Dev Biol 2016;5(1):5–23.

Update on Fibrocartilaginous Disease Clinical Examination

Michelle L. Butterworth, DPM, FACFAS*,
Alan J. Block, DPM, MS, FACFAS

KEYWORDS

- Fibrocartilaginous disease • Plantar plate • Achilles tendon • Clinical examination

PLANTAR PLATE DISORDERS

The plantar plate may be a small anatomic structure but when damaged, it can contribute to significant pathology and result in complex deformities. The treatment of plantar plate disorders is challenging even for the best foot and ankle surgeons and it is often a topic of significant debate. Before treatment is instilled, however, an accurate diagnosis must be made. The diagnosis of plantar plate dysfunction is difficult and is highly dependent on the clinical examination and a high index of suspicion. The authors review demographics, patient history, causative factors, differential diagnosis, physical examination, clinical tests, and radiographic evaluation for plantar plate dysfunction.

Plantar plate dysfunction typically begins as attrition and distention of the joint. If left untreated it can progress to partial tearing or complete rupture of the plantar plate. This creates instability of the lesser metatarsophalangeal joint (MTPJ) and sagittal plane and frequently transverse plane subluxation and dislocation occurs with subsequent digital deformity (**Fig. 1**). Coughlin,[1] in 1987, coined the term "second crossover toe" to describe this lesser MTPJ instability. Although the second toe is most commonly involved, other digits have also been reported with this same clinical entity.[2–5] In 1995, Yu and Judge[6] described a specific syndrome associated with lesser MTPJ pathology and termed it predislocation syndrome (PDS). Yu and colleagues[6,7] then developed a classification system for PDS based on clinical findings:

Stage I: Mild edema dorsally and plantarly, extreme tenderness plantar and distal to the joint, and no anatomic malalignment (**Fig. 2**).
Stage II: Moderate edema with noticeable deviation of the digit clinically and radiographically, and there is lack of toe purchase (**Fig. 3**).

Williamsburg Foot Center, 308 Logan Street, Kingstree, SC 29556, USA
* Corresponding author.
E-mail address: mbutter@ftc.net

Clin Podiatr Med Surg 39 (2022) 371–392
https://doi.org/10.1016/j.cpm.2022.03.002
0891-8422/22/© 2022 Elsevier Inc. All rights reserved.

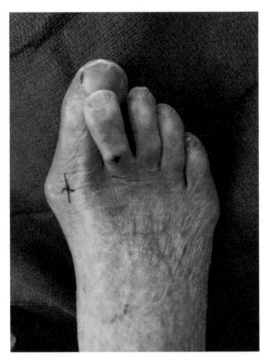

Fig. 1. Classic clinical presentation of plantar plate dysfunction. The second toe is subluxated dorsally and medially and lies dorsally on the hallux.

Stage III: Moderate edema with pronounced deviation clinically, and subluxation or dislocation on radiographs (**Fig. 4**).

Demographics and Patient History

Coughlin[3] recognized two different populations at risk for developing second MTPJ instability. One group was sedentary, older women aged 50 to 70 years old, with a

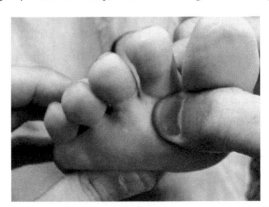

Fig. 2. Clinical examination showing stage I of PDS. There is localized edema plantarly and tenderness to palpation of the plantar lateral aspect of the second metatarsophalangeal joint. No digital malalignment is seen.

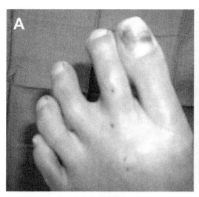
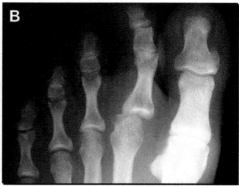

Fig. 3. (*A*) Clinical examination showing stage II of PDS. There is medial deviation of the second toe resulting in gapping between the second and third toes. (*B*) Radiograph showing stage II of PDS. There is obvious medial deviation of the second metatarsophalangeal joint.

prevalent use of high-heeled shoes. The second group was predominantly athletic men aged 25 to 64 years, with repetitive activity causing the joint instability. So, although lesser MTPJ instability is more prevalent in the female population, the same process has also been reported in younger male athletes.[3,8] The typical patient profile in the authors experience, however, is a middle-aged female more commonly than male, with an acute or subacute onset of pain about the plantar aspect of the lesser MTPJ. There is typically no history of trauma or injury. The patient may describe an active lifestyle including walking, running, or aerobics or a recent increase in activity. The patient's discomfort is often times described as an aching or throbbing and sometimes sharp pain, which is increased with activity. They may also relate the feeling of a lump or bruise on the ball of their foot. Of significance is the magnitude of pain relayed by the patient is usually markedly out of proportion from what is appreciated on the physical examination. There may also be some anxiety and even depression present in these patients, because this condition often significantly interferes with their activities and lifestyle. The patient may have even sought treatment previously, but the condition may have been misdiagnosed or treatments failed to resolve their symptoms.

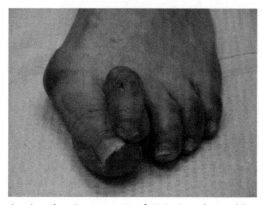

Fig. 4. Clinical examination showing stage III of PDS. Complete subluxation of the second metatarsophalangeal joint has resulted.

Causative Factors

PDS can best be described as a monoarticular synovitis or capsulitis that creates attenuation of the plantar plate. Both intrinsic and extrinsic factors are the cause of this entity.[1,9] Intrinsic factors, such as inflammatory arthropathies, including rheumatoid arthritis and connective tissue disorders, have been reported to result in lesser MTPJ instability.[10] The capsular distention created by these disorders leads to deterioration of the joint and subsequent attrition of the plantar plate. Acute trauma has also been reported as a factor in plantar plate attenuation and tearing and lesser MTPJ instability (**Fig. 5**).[11]

More frequently, however, the cause of PDS is more insidious and results from extrinsic factors including abnormal biomechanics and structural deformities.[12,13] Any force that creates increased and/or abnormal loading on the forefoot can cause lesser MTPJ instability.[14]

First ray insufficiency, including medial column hypermobility and an elongated or elevated first metatarsal, can result in increased lateral loading and subsequent lesser MTPJ instability. Hallux abducto valgus deformities can cause lateral deviation of the hallux onto the second toe and cause retrograde buckling of the second toe and subluxation of the MTPJ (**Fig. 6**). An elongated metatarsal can also cause increased stress across the MTPJ resulting in synovitis/capsulitis and attenuation of the plantar plate (**Fig. 7**). One study reported 80% of patients with MTPJ subluxation had a long second metatarsal.[1] Hindfoot deformities including pes planovalgus, pes cavus, and equinus are also common contributing factors to lesser MTPJ instability and digital deformities. Of course, shoe gear that creates increased pressure and stress on the forefoot, such as high-heeled shoes and shoes with heels lifts, can cause instability of the lesser MTPJs and plantar plate dysfunction.

Differential Diagnosis

A delay in the evaluation and treatment of plantar plate disorders is common because of the insidious onset of pain and deformity. Plantar plate dysfunction does not always result in immediate pain. This can contribute to misdiagnosis and delay of care. An

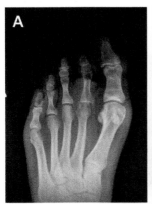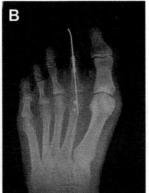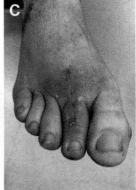

Fig. 5. (A) Acute, traumatic dorsal and medial dislocation of the second metatarsophalangeal joint with rupture of the plantar plate following a fall. (B) Postoperative radiograph after repair of the plantar plate, second metatarsal osteotomy, and second hammertoe repair. (C) Postoperative photograph showing good alignment and reduction with procedures performed.

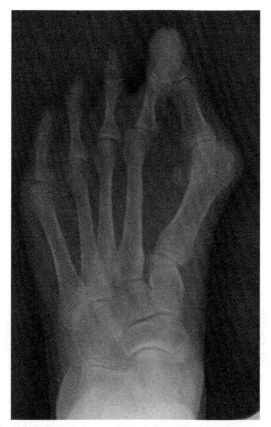

Fig. 6. Radiograph with hallux abductovalgus deformity. The hallux is abutting the second toe causing retrograde buckling and subluxation of the second metatarsophalangeal joint. Patient also has an elongated second metatarsal.

accurate diagnosis is paramount so that treatment is instilled promptly, so that the progression of the plantar plate insufficiency is halted and tearing and rupture of the plantar plate and joint dislocation and deformity are prevented. Frequently, however, patients become concerned only after progression of the deformity has become severe and a fixed hammertoe has developed.[2] In studies conducted by Nery and colleagues,[5] the number of patients with grade 3 or 4 plantar plate tears was larger than the number of patients with grade 1 or 2 tears. This finding suggests that the condition is not frequently diagnosed until the deformity and symptoms have progressed to a more severe level.[5]

Metatarsalgia is a common term used to describe generalized forefoot pain, and MTPJ instability is one of the most common causes for this condition. PDS is primarily a diagnosis of exclusion and clinical suspicion is one of the best tools for early diagnosis. The differential diagnosis for PDS should include metatarsal stress fracture, intermetatarsal neuroma, degenerative arthritis, systemic arthritis, synovitis/capsulitis, synovial cyst formation, and Freiberg infarction.

Because neuroma symptoms closely mimic the symptoms of PDS, differentiating these two entities is challenging. Patients with an interdigital neuroma, however, typically have symptoms including tingling or burning, and possibly radiating pain or even

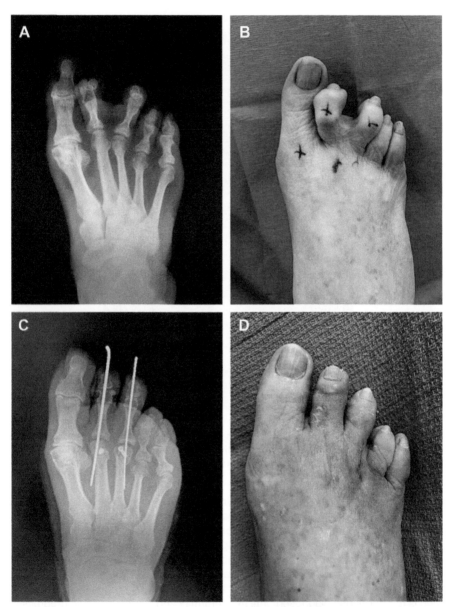

Fig. 7. (*A*) Radiographs of a 78-year-old woman with elongated second and third metatarsals and gapping between the second and third toes. Cortical thickening of the second metatarsal is also seen. (*B*) Preoperative clinical presentation of the hammertoe deformities and the metatarsophalangeal joint dislocation after failure of the plantar plates. (*C*) Postoperative radiograph after plantar plate repair, transitional metatarsal osteotomies, and hammertoe repair. (*D*) Good clinical alignment and reduction of deformities with the chosen procedures.

numbness into the toes. MTPJ instability, however, usually does not present with these neuritic-type symptoms unless there is a concomitant neuroma. Also, with MTPJ instability, compression of the transverse metatarsal arch does not usually illicit the typical "Mulder click" as it does when an interdigital neuroma is present. According to Coughlin and colleagues,[15] there is the presence of a concomitant interdigital neuroma in nearly 20% of patients with lesser MTPJ instability. The use of a local anesthetic as a diagnostic block along the digital nerve in the suspected interspace can aid in differentiating interdigital neuroma from PDS. If the symptoms are relieved with the nerve block, then an interdigital neuroma is most likely present. A patient with MTPJ instability and plantar plate dysfunction, however, usually has continued pain at the MTPJ after the nerve block. Although this diagnostic tool is helpful, it is not always consistent, and the physician must rely on a high degree of clinical suspicion and a focused history and physical examination to diagnose plantar plate dysfunction.

Physical Examination

On physical examination, a patient with plantar plate dysfunction typically has exquisite tenderness of the lesser MTPJ that is disproportionate to any other objective clinical findings. Although originally described as unique to the second MTPJ,[1] in a large series by Nery and colleagues[5] a total of 55 plantar plate tears were observed with two-thirds of them involving the second MTPJ and one-third involving either the third or fourth MTPJ.

The focal area of tenderness to palpation of the MTPJ is plantar and just distal to the metatarsal head at the insertion of the plantar plate apparatus on the base of the proximal phalanx. This is thought to result from bursitis or inflammation of the plantar plate.[16] If transverse plane deformity is present, the pain is typically more profound on the plantar lateral aspect of the joint with medial deviation of the toe and on the plantar medial aspect of the joint with lateral deviation of the toe (**Fig. 8**). Range of motion of the lesser MTPJ is typically painful, especially with plantarflexion.[17] Decreased motion of the joint is common, either from the inflammation of the joint itself or secondary to patient guarding. Joint crepitus, however, is usually absent. Also, active flexion and extension of the toe is usually not compromised. Mild localized edema is also usually present secondary to capsular distention. The edema plantarly is usually obvious but the edema dorsally may only be noticed by obliteration of the normal extensor tendon contours. Mild increased warmth may also be present.

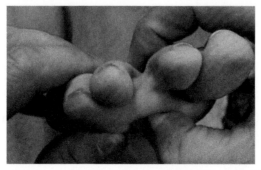

Fig. 8. On clinical examination, there is medial deviation of the second toe and tenderness to palpation of the plantar lateral aspect of the second metatarsophalangeal joint.

In the early phase of PDS, typically there is little or no malalignment of the MTPJ and a hammertoe deformity is often absent. As the plantar plate dysfunction progresses, however, subluxation/dislocation of the MTPJ and subsequent digital deformity typically result. In most cases, however, even in the early stages of PDS, weightbearing stance demonstrates subtle malalignment of the involved digit with some loss of toe purchase. One may even notice mild gapping between the affected toe and adjacent toe (**Fig. 9**). During gait, pain is most common during the propulsive phase, and is debilitating. Also, the patient may unconsciously be splinting the area of pain and walking on the outside of their foot. This may contribute to other areas of compensatory pain more proximal in the foot and ankle. As the deformity progresses, the toe continues to subluxate dorsally and a hammertoe deformity typically results. Transverse plane malalignment with medial deviation at the MTPJ can result, and with continued progression of the plantar plate dysfunction the dreaded crossover toe can result, signaling the end stage of the syndrome (**Fig. 10**). Transverse plane malalignment, with lateral deviation at the MTPJ, can also result, but is less common. It is important to remember that the lesser digits and MTPJs typically move in a herdlike fashion, so when one dislocates, often the others follow resulting in multiple deformities (**Fig. 11**).

Clinical Tests

Lachman test is the most common test used to evaluate MTPJ instability and the structural integrity of the plantar plate. Defined by Thompson and Hamilton,[18] it has also been referred to as the dorsal drawer test and the vertical stress test. This test

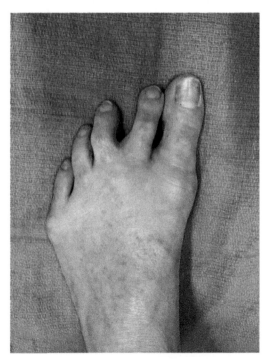

Fig. 9. The plantar plate is attenuated in this patient as seen by some medial deviation of the second toe and gapping between the second and third toes.

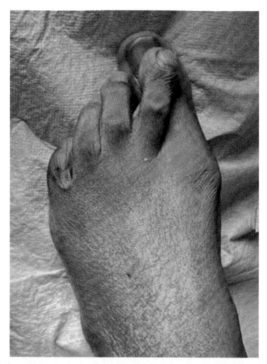

Fig. 10. Failure of the plantar plate resulting in a crossover second toe.

is performed by stabilizing the metatarsal with one hand and then grasping the proximal phalanx with the other hand. A vertical stress, in a dorsally oriented direction, is then applied to the proximal phalanx. To perform the test accurately, the physician must ensure that the force applied on the proximal phalanx is purely vertical and not dorsiflexion at the MTPJ. A positive test is described as greater than 50% of dorsal displacement of the proximal phalanx in the vertical height of the metatarsal head, or 2 mm of dorsal displacement of the proximal phalanx (**Fig. 12**). A positive test is pathognomonic for plantar plate attenuation or tear[8] and usually reproduces the patient's pain. Often, the examiner can actually feel the MTPJ subluxate or dislocate in the presence of a plantar plate tear.

The paper pullout test is another common clinical modality used to aid in the diagnosis of plantar plate dysfunction. It was described by Bouche and Heit[12] and can measure digital purchase and assess the plantarflexion strength of the digit. With the patient standing, a strip of paper is placed underneath the tip of the affected digit. While the patient plantarflexes the toe to grasp the paper, the examiner pulls the paper out from beneath the toe. A positive test is seen when the paper is successfully removed with little or no resistance (**Fig. 13**).

Radiographic Evaluation

The diagnosis of lesser MTPJ instability and plantar plate dysfunction is established primarily based on subjective complaints and clinical findings. Radiographs can assist in confirming the clinical diagnosis, by ruling out other entities within the differential diagnosis and evaluating osseous pathology present.

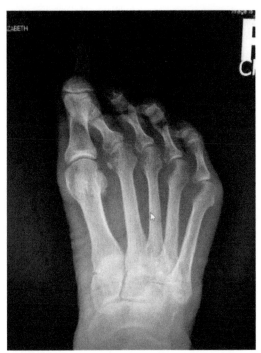

Fig. 11. Radiograph showing medial subluxation of all of the lesser metatarsophalangeal joints. When one joint subluxates, it is common for the other joints to follow the same course.

Standard weight-bearing radiographic examination of the affected foot should be used to assess osseous pathology, joint congruity, angular deformity, and intraarticular changes.[8] The integrity of the plantar plate is evaluated by the alignment of the MTPJ and the position of the toe on the anteroposterior and lateral radiographs. These views assist the physician in recognizing the full degree of the deformity and subluxation of the MTPJ in the sagittal and transverse planes. Incongruency of the joint space is appreciated as the digit deviates in the sagittal and transverse planes. The normal clear space of the lesser MTPJ is 2 to 3 mm, and the joint surfaces should be congruent.[4] When dorsal subluxation occurs, the clear space is obliterated as the concave base of the proximal phalanx migrates dorsally over the convex metatarsal head (**Fig. 14**).

The anteroposterior radiograph can also be used to assess any abnormal metatarsal length patterns that might contribute to the development and progression of the deformity. The length assessment is done by drawing a line connecting the distal articular surface of the first and third metatarsals, and then measuring the protrusion of the second metatarsal beyond this line. A positive value indicates an excessive second metatarsal length. Coughlin[4] noted that patients with clinical joint instability had elongated second metatarsals and cortical hypertrophy in approximately 50% of involved second metatarsals. Cortical hypertrophy is determined by measuring the medial and lateral diaphyseal cortex of the second metatarsal shaft and comparing it with the third. Cortical thickening is often a sign of metatarsal overload, and one should always evaluate for a possible stress fracture as part of the differential diagnosis.

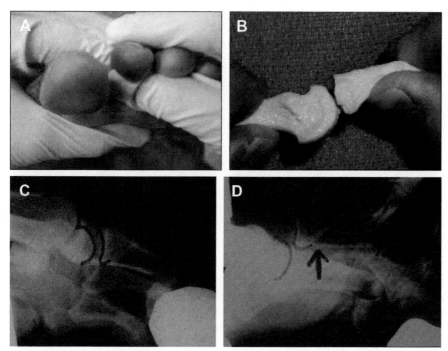

Fig. 12. (*A, B*) The vertical stress test is performed clinically and then demonstrated on saw bones. It is imperative that the force applied on the proximal phalanx is purely vertical and the movement is not dorsiflexion of the metatarsophalangeal joint. (*C, D*) Radiographs of a positive vertical stress test, indicative of attenuation or a tear of the plantar plate. Notice that there is greater than 50% of dorsal displacement of the proximal phalanx in the vertical height of the metatarsal head.

The most reliable radiographic indicator of second MTPJ instability is the angle of the second MTPJ in relationship to the hallux and third MTPJ angle. In a retrospective study, Kaz and Coughlin[8] demonstrated that the second MTPJ angle was significantly higher in the bunion group than the nonbunion group. They also found a significant relationship between a crossover second toe deformity and the length of the second metatarsal, metatarsal cortex thickness, and radiographic measurement of deformities including pes planovalgus, metatarsus adductus, and metatarsus primus elevatus.

Radiographic evaluation should also be used to assess intraarticular degenerative changes. Although it is not common in the early stages of plantar plate dysfunction, degeneration of the joint can result from long-standing joint malposition and chronic dorsal subluxation of the proximal phalanx with impaction on the metatarsal head. It is important to differentiate plantar plate dysfunction from Freiberg infarction and other arthritic entities.

Radiographic examination should be performed on all patients with suspected plantar plate dysfunction, but it should be used as an adjunct to rule out other entities in the differential diagnosis, and not used to make the diagnosis of plantar plate pathology, because findings are inconsistent. Radiographs can indicate a lesser MTPJ planal deformity, but they do not provide conclusive evidence regarding the role of the plantar plate. A high index of suspicion and thorough clinical evaluation is warranted for a conclusive diagnosis. Other imaging modalities, such as ultrasound and

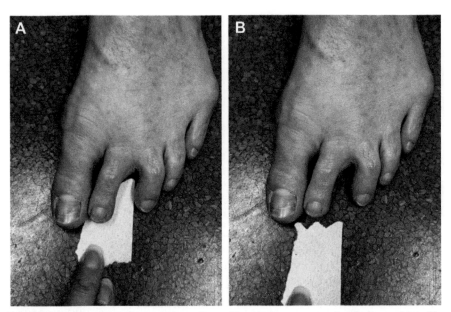

Fig. 13. (*A*) The paper pullout test is performed by placing paper under the second toe. The patient plantarflexes and grips down on the paper. (*B*) The paper is easily removed with no resistance indicating a positive paper pullout test and lack of toe purchase consistent with plantar plate dysfunction.

MRI, can assist in establishing a diagnosis and have been used to isolate and visualize plantar plate tears. These modalities are discussed in full detail elsewhere in this issue.

Summary

Lesser MTPJ instability is a challenging entity for the foot and ankle surgeon. A correct diagnosis is crucial to instill an appropriate treatment plan that results in a successful outcome and a satisfied patient. The diagnosis of plantar plate dysfunction depends on subjective complaints, physical examination, and clinical tests. Radiographs can aid in evaluating osseous pathology and joint alignment and integrity, but is mostly used for ruling out other entities in the differential diagnosis. For such a small anatomic structure, when it is damaged, plantar plate dysfunction can result in significant and complex deformities. Because the plantar plate is primarily composed of type I collagen, it is unlikely that a tear spontaneously heals with time.[19–21] For this reason, it is of the utmost importance to have a proper diagnosis as early as possible so that treatment can be used. The surgeon, therefore, should always have a high index of suspicion of potential plantar plate pathology when lesser MTPJ symptoms present. Although conservative measures can temporarily relieve the pain of an unstable lesser MTPJ, they do not correct deformity.[2–4] A good clinical examination results in a correct diagnosis so that the physician can provide a proper treatment plan that it is hoped prevents resultant deformity.

INSERTIONAL ACHILLES DISORDERS

The Achilles tendon is the longest, thickest, and strongest tendon in the human body. It is enveloped in a thin vascularized paratenon. The tendon itself, however, is largely avascular, especially in the midportion. This lack of vascular perfusion renders the

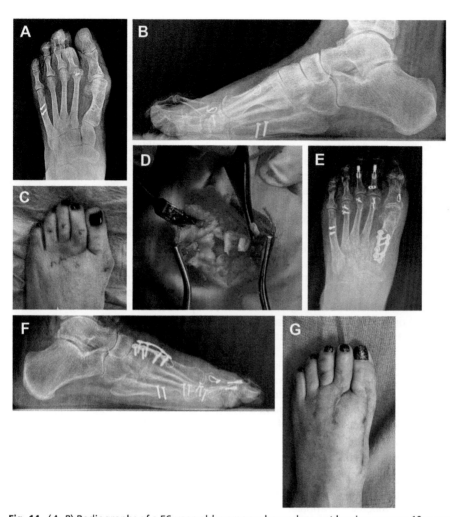

Fig. 14. (*A, B*) Radiographs of a 56-year-old woman who underwent bunion surgery 10 years prior and then plantar plate repair and second metatarsal osteotomy 3 years ago. She states her foot was good until she fell recently and traumatically dislocated her second metatarsophalangeal joint. Dorsal and lateral dislocation is obvious, with no space seen in the second metatarsophalangeal joint. A recurrent hallux abductovalgus deformity is also noted. (*C*) Clinical photograph to correlate with the previous radiographs. (*D*) Intraoperative picture showing rupture of both the plantar plate and the flexor tendon. (*E, F*) Postoperative radiographs showing good reduction of deformities with the procedures performed. There was minimal plantar plate available for repair; therefore, it was sutured into the base of the proximal phalanx and held in place with a metal button. The second metatarsophalangeal joint is now in good alignment but there is some degenerative changes from the previous surgeries and injury. (*G*) Postoperative photograph showing good digital alignment.

Achilles tendon highly susceptible to injury and pathology with poor healing potential.[22] A thorough history and physical examination, therefore, is crucial to make an accurate diagnosis and initiate proper management. Mismanaged or neglected injuries and pathology can markedly decrease a patient's quality of life.

Demographics and Patient History

Disorders of the Achilles tendon are common in active and sedentary persons, but they are more common in athletes and those playing recreational sports.[23] Among athletes, the lifetime prevalence of chronic tendinopathy is 23.9% compared with 2.1% in the general population.[24] Achilles tendinosis accounts for 10% of all running injuries.[25] Achilles tendinopathy is also common among athletes participating in racquet sports, volleyball, and soccer.[26] There is also a genetic predilection that can significantly increase the incidence of Achilles tendinosis.[27] Many systemic etiologies including diabetes, seronegative spondyloarthropathies, gout, and rheumatoid arthritis can also predispose a patient to Achilles tendon disorders.

A thorough problem-focused history should include specific details of the inciting event when pain began, the presence and duration of prodromal symptoms, usual daily activities including any athletic activity, any new activities started, any history of injury and trauma, and any treatment rendered including medications and injections. A complete medical history is also important, taking special note of any of the systemic etiologies listed previously.

Patients with insertional Achilles tendon disorders typically complain of pain that is increased with weight bearing and activities. They may often relate poststatic dyskinesia. Commonly, patients have a history of changes in activity level. They may have had a period of inactivity and have recently started a new walking or running regimen or a new exercise program. Walking on a treadmill, especially on an incline, can increase stress on the Achilles tendon making it prone to injury. In runners, a large percentage of injuries may be associated with a change in training conditions including a sudden increase in mileage.[28] Pain at the onset of running may be followed by a period of relief after sufficient warm-up but then the pain returns as the activity increases. Although Achilles tendon disorders commonly result from athletic overuse injuries, up to one-third of the people affected are nonathletic, middle-aged, overweight patients with no history of increased physical activity.[29]

Causative Factors

Although several theories exist, the cause of insertional Achilles tendon disorders still remains unclear and is multifactorial. Proposed theories include overuse, poor tissue vascularity, mechanical imbalances of the extremity, and genetic predisposition.[30,31] Many causative factors have been implicated including intrinsic and extrinsic sources. Achilles tendinopathy secondary to overuse is thought to arise from repetitive microtrauma in the central portion of the tendon.[32] This is common with intrinsic factors that are biomechanical in nature. These can occur when there is high physical stress placed on the insertion of the Achilles tendon in the presence of pathology, such as gastrocsoleus or gastrocnemius equinus, pes cavus, pes valgus, excessive frontal plane motion of the rearfoot, compensated forefoot varus, and lateral ankle instability.

Age, sex, and body weight and height are some other intrinsic factors that have been shown to play a role in Achilles tendon pathology. A retrospective study, by Holmes and Lin,[33] identified several patient factors that were more likely to be associated with Achilles tendinopathy. These included hypertension, diabetes, obesity, and a previous exposure to steroids or estrogen. Each of these factors has the potential to decrease the microvascularity of tendons; therefore, it was postulated that they may play a role in the development of Achilles tendon pathology.[33] Other studies have found advancing age, previous injury, exposure to quinolone antibiotics, and endocrine and metabolic abnormalities to be associated with Achilles tendon disorders.[34,35]

Changes in training patterns, poor technique, previous injuries, footwear, and environmental factors, such as training on hard floors or slippery or slanted surfaces, are extrinsic factors that may predispose one to Achilles tendon dysfunction.[36] Excessive loading of tendons during vigorous physical training is regarded as the main pathologic stimulus for Achilles tendinopathy.[37]

Differential Diagnosis

The diagnosis of insertional Achilles tendon disorders is easy. This group of disorders includes all the entities resulting from posterior heel pain at the Achilles tendon insertion site. The difficult part in the diagnosis is identifying the proper disorder and using the proper terminology. Most authorities advocate the use of the term "tendinopathy" to encompass each of the subclasses of Achilles tendon pathology including peritendinitis, tendinitis, and tendinosis. These terms are commonly used when discussing Achilles tendon disorders, and unfortunately, they are often used interchangeably. It is important for the physician to understand the difference between the entities to render an accurate diagnosis so proper treatment is instilled.

Achilles peritendinitis denotes a generalized inflammation involving the tissues surrounding the Achilles tendon, yet without affecting the tendon itself. Achilles tendinitis is an acute inflammatory reaction that is typically short term with proper treatment. Achilles tendinosis, however, is a degenerative process with deterioration of the tendon fibers. It is typically more challenging to treat, and often results in more long-term effects. Underestimation of the chronic degenerative nature of tendinosis can lead to long-term disability; therefore, the differentiation between acute tendinitis is critical.[29]

Other possible diagnoses for posterior heel pain includes retrocalcaneal bursitis, neuritis, and retrocalcaneal exostosis. All of these may be present in addition to the actual tendon pathology. Increased tension on the insertion site of the Achilles tendon on the posterior heel can cause inflammation and increased pressure on the bursa leading to bursitis. The localized inflammation can also cause irritation to the surrounding nerve causing neuritis. Finally, this physical strain on the insertion site of the Achilles tendon can lead to the development of a degenerative process in the anterior aspect of the Achilles tendon. This anterior portion of the tendon undergoes endochondral ossification at its insertion because of the physical stress and degenerative process. This ossification results in the enthesis or retrocalcaneal exostosis (**Fig. 15**).[38] Benjamin and colleagues[39] described the exostosis developing as a way for the bone to have a greater surface area on the tendon.

Although it is easy for the physician to have tunnel vision when it comes to posterior heel pain, they must rule out other potential, but less likely, diagnoses including, but not limited to, stress fractures, soft tissue and bone tumors, tarsal tunnel, arthropathy, and infection. A thorough history and physical examination and standard radiographs remain the cornerstone of an accurate diagnosis. Advanced imaging, such as MRI, can also be performed if needed.

Physical Examination

Most insertional Achilles tendon disorders are diagnosed on a clinical basis. On examination, the patient typically has pain directly over the posterior heel at the Achilles tendon insertion site where an osseous prominence is present. The physician should palpate the entire length of the Achilles tendon to feel for fullness, irregularity, gapping, and tenderness. This should be performed on both lower extremities for comparison. The tendon insertion on the affected side commonly appears thicker than a normal tendon insertion (**Fig. 16**).

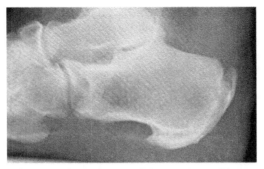

Fig. 15. Radiograph of a retrocalcaneal exostosis in a patient with posterior heel pain. The osseous spur spans the entire posterior calcaneus from medial to lateral.

Localized edema is also usually present and can become quite noticeable when compared with the contralateral extremity. Often the area is so painful and edematous, patients cannot wear a closed-back shoe. Occasionally, erythema and increased warmth of the area are present secondary to the localized inflammation (**Fig. 17**). Because insertional Achilles tendinitis typically presents in the absence of trauma, ecchymosis is usually not present. Crepitus on examination is indicative of peritendinits where fibrous exudate fills the tendon sheath. When the ankle is put though a

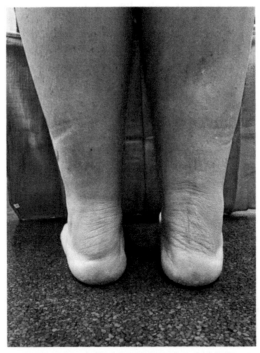

Fig. 16. Clinical presentation of a patient with insertional Achilles tendonitis on her left side. Notice the thickening of the tendon and localized edema compared with her right side, which has already undergone surgical intervention.

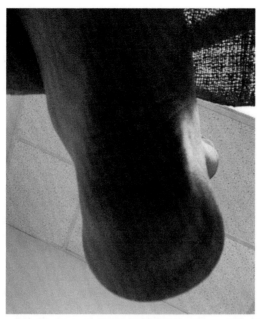

Fig. 17. Erythema, edema, and increased warmth is seen in this patient with Achilles tendonitis consistent with the acute inflammatory process of this disorder.

range of motion, the area of pain with peritendinitis does not change or move with the tendon.

Range of motion of the rearfoot and ankle joints, manual muscle testing, and gait analysis should also be performed. Pain may be present with passive and active dorsiflexion of the ankle. Weakness of the gastrocsoleus complex is commonly seen rendering the patient unable to perform a single-legged heel raise on the affected extremity. Patients usually have an antalgic gait with early heel off.

Retrocalcaneal exostoses are commonly present with insertional Achilles tendon disorders. These osseous spurs are the source of significant pain and can be large and lie within the Achilles tendon (**Fig. 18**). It has been documented, however, that these exostoses are as common on the asymptomatic side as they are on the

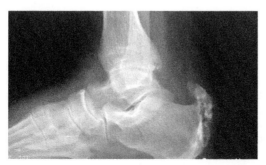

Fig. 18. Radiograph showing a large retrocalcaneal exostosis that has extended superiorly above the border of the calcaneus and is also intratendinous. This patient had significant pain and was unable to wear any closed-back shoes.

symptomatic side.[38–40] A correlation has been made, however, between a large exostosis being symptomatic and a small exostosis on the contralateral limb being asymptomatic.[40,41] An area of osseous prominence may also be palpated just proximal to the Achilles tendon insertion site if a coexisting Haglund deformity is present.

The physician should also examine the patient for other pathologies and sources of pain besides from the tendon itself. If pain is produced on squeezing the soft tissue between the Achilles tendon and the posterior calcaneus, a retrocalcaneal bursitis may be present. This is usually a deep, chronic pain. Patients may also complain of localized numbness or paresthesias secondary to nerve compression from the surrounding inflammation and tendon pathology.

The physician must also evaluate the patient for underlying deformities predisposing the patient to this Achilles tendon pathology including equinus, pes planovalgus, pes cavus, and lateral ankle instability. Equinus, caused by gastrocnemius contracture, has been well documented as being associated with the development of Achilles tendinopathy.[42–44] On the contrary, Mahieu and colleagues[45] in a prospective study found that decreased plantarflexion strength and an increased amount of dorsiflexion were significant predictors of Achilles tendon overuse injuries.[45]

Clinical Tests

There are a couple of helpful clinical tests the physician can perform to complete a thorough evaluation of the patient and render an accurate diagnosis of insertional Achilles tendon pathology. The arc sign is used to evaluate tendon thickening and can help distinguish between tendon and paratenon lesions. The tendon is palpated while the patient actively dorsiflexes and plantarflexes the ankle. A positive arc sign is present when the swelling or thickening is visualized to move relative to the malleoli during the active movement. This is typically indicative of tendon degeneration.[46] If the thickened portion is not observed to move with the active range of motion, it is thought that peritendinitis is present.

The Royal London Hospital test is performed by palpating the tendon to identify the area of local tenderness while the ankle is initially in neutral position. The patient then actively dorsiflexes and plantarflexes the ankle. A positive finding is when palpation of the tender area of the tendon at rest results in significantly less or no pain at the same location when the ankle is maximally dorsiflexed.[46]

Although these clinical tests are helpful and aid in making a diagnosis of insertional Achilles tendon pathology, a single test or finding should not be relied on independently for a definitive diagnosis. The physician should rely on a full history and physical examination and imaging modalities, when needed, for a final assessment.

Radiographic Evaluation

Although radiographs are typically not the imaging modality of choice for tendon pathology, it still has a role in thoroughly evaluating insertional Achilles tendon pathology and should be performed on all patients with posterior heel pain. Radiographs aid in diagnosing associated osseous abnormalities and concomitant structural deformities, and they can also aid in eliminating other potential diagnoses, such as stress fractures or bone tumors.

Lateral and calcaneal axial radiographs are typically the most helpful views when assessing posterior heel pathology. Osseous irregularities are frequently observed at the insertion of the Achilles tendon with osseous spurring. These posterior osteophytes can range from very small to very large and usually span the width of the posterior calcaneus (**Fig. 19**). Intratendinous ossification may also be seen (**Fig. 20**). Other osseous irregularities, including Haglund deformity, can also be identified on standard

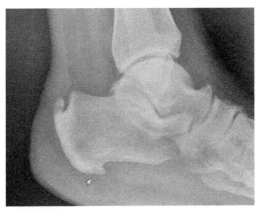

Fig. 19. Retrocalcaneal exostosis spanning the entire posterior calcaneus. A Haglund deformity is also present with prominence of the posterior superior aspect of the calcaneus.

radiographs. Kager triangle is evaluated from the lateral radiograph. Obscurity of Kager triangle typically indicates that a retrocalcaneal bursitis is present.[47] Structural deformities and osseous alignment should also be assessed radiographically because these may be contributing factors in the Achilles tendon pathology. The calcaneal axial view can aid in determining the presence of calcaneal varus and the positioning of the exostosis if present. An increase in the calcaneal inclination angle, seen on the lateral view, has been linked to insertional tendinosis; however, Shibuya and colleagues[48] refuted this assumption stating that there is no statistical difference in the calcaneal inclination angle in those that have exostoses and those that do not.

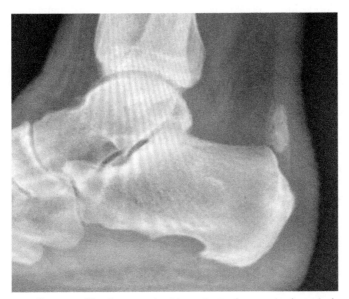

Fig. 20. Intratendinous ossification seen in this patient who required surgical removal for pain relief.

Other imaging studies, including ultrasound and MRI, may be useful in assessing tendon pathology and further discussions regarding these modalities is provided elsewhere in this issue.

Summary

Insertional Achilles tendon disorders are common among active and inactive patients. There is also a high predilection for Achilles tendon pathology among athletes. Although the diagnosis of these injuries is usually easy, the treatment is challenging. Therefore, it is paramount to make an accurate diagnosis and identify the exact Achilles pathology present. Treatment protocols can differ depending on the amount and degree of tendon involvement. A clinical examination and thorough history are therefore critical for an accurate assessment and implementation of a proper treatment plan to provide the best outcome for the patient.

DISCLOSURE

The authors have nothing to disclose.

REFERENCES

1. Coughlin MJ. Crossover second toe deformity. Foot Ankle 1987;8:29.
2. Coughlin MJ. When to suspect crossover second toe deformity. J Musculoskel Med 1987;4:39–48.
3. Coughlin MJ. Second metatarsophalangeal joint instability in the athlete. Foot Ankle 1993;14:309–19.
4. Coughlin MJ. Subluxation and dislocation of the second metatarsophalangeal joint. Orthop Clin North Am 1989;20:535–51.
5. Nery C, Coughlin MJ, Baumfeld D, et al. Lesser metatarsophalangeal joint instability: prospective evaluation and repair of plantar plate and capsular insufficiency. Foot Ankle Int 2012;33:301–11.
6. Yu GV, Judge MS. Predislocation syndrome of the lesser metatarsophalangeal joint: a distinct clinical entity. In: Camasta CA, Vickers NS, Carter Sr, editors. Reconstructive surgery of the foot and leg: update '95. Tucker (GA): The Podiatry Institute; 1995. p. 109–13.
7. Yu GV, Judge MS, Hudson JR, et al. Predislocation syndrome: progression subluxation/dislocation of the lesser metatarsophalangeal joint. J Am Podiatr Med Assoc 2002;92:182–99.
8. Kaz AJ, Coughlin MJ. Crossover second toe: demographics, etiology, and radiographic assessment. Foot Ankle Int 2007;28:1223–37.
9. Mendicino RW, Statler TK, Saltrick KR, et al. Predislocation syndrome: a review and retrospective analysis of eight patients. J Foot Ankle Surg 2001;40(4):214–24.
10. Mann RA, Coughlin MJ. The rheumatoid foot: review of literature and method of treatment. Orthop Rev 1979;8:105–12.
11. Brunet JA, Tubin S. Traumatic dislocations of the lesser toes. Foot Ankle Int 1997;18:406–11.
12. Bouche RT, Heit EJ. Combined plantar plate and hammertoe repair with flexor digitorum longus tendon transfer for chronic, severe sagittal plane instability of the lesser metatarsophalangeal joints: preliminary observations. J Foot Ankle Surg 2008;47:125–37.
13. Mann RA, Mizel MS. Monoarticular nontraumatic synovitis of the metatarsophalangeal joint: a new diagnosis? Foot Ankle 1985;6:18–21.

14. Butterworth M. Tendon transfers for management of digital and lesser metatarso-phalangeal joint deformities. Clin Podiatr Med Surg 2016;33(1):71–84.
15. Coughlin MJ, Schenck RC, Shumas PS, et al. Concurrent interdigital neuroma and MTP joint instability: long term results and treatment. Foot Ankle Int 2002;23:1018–25.
16. Fishco WD. The sub-two syndrome. In: Miller SJ, Mahan KT, YU GV, et al, editors. Reconstructive surgery of the foot and leg: update '98. Tucker (GA): The Podiatry Institute; 1998. p. 107–11.
17. Root ML, Orien WP, Weed JH. Normal and abnormal function of the foot. Los Angeles (CA): Clinical Biomechanics Corp; 1977. p. 218.
18. Thompson FM, Hamilton WG. Problems of the second metatarsophalangeal joint. Orthopedics 1987;10:83–9.
19. Deland JT, Lee KT, Sobel M, et al. Anatomy of the plantar plate and its attachments in the lesser metatarsophalangeal joint. Foot Ankle Int 1995;16:480–6.
20. Powless SH, Elze ME. Metatarsophalangeal joint capsule tears: an analysis by arthrography, a new classification system and surgical management. J Foot Ankle Surg 2001;40:374–89.
21. Johnston RB III, Smith J, Daniels T. The plantar plate of the lesser toes: an anatomical study in human cadavers. Foot Ankle Int 1994;15:276–82.
22. Chen TM, Rozen WM, Pan WR, et al. The arterial anatomy of the Achilles tendon: anatomical study and clinical applications. Clin Anat 2009;22(3):377–85.
23. Alfredson H, Lorentzon R. Chronic Achilles tendinosis: recommendations for treatment and prevention. Sports Med 2000;29(2):135–46.
24. Kujala UM, Sarna S, Kaprio J. Cumulative incidence of Achilles tendon rupture and tendinopathy in male former elite athletes. Clin J Sport Med 2005;15(3):133–5.
25. Francis P, Whatman C, Sheerin K, et al. The proportion of lower limb running injuries by gender, anatomical location, and specific pathology: a systematic review. J Sports Sci Med 2019;18(1):21–31.
26. Maffulli N, Binfield PM, King JB. Tendon problems in athletic individuals. J Bone Joint Surg Am 1998;80:142–4.
27. Kraemer R, Wuerfel W, Lorenzen J, et al. Analysis of hereditary and medical risk factors in Achilles tendinopathy and Achilles tendon ruptures: a matched pair analysis. Arch Orthop Trauma Surg 2012;132(6):847–53.
28. Clancy Wg, Neidhart D, Brand RL. Achilles tendinitis in runners: a report of five cases. Am J Sports Med 1976;4:46–57.
29. Maffulli N, Khan KM, Puddu G. Overuse tendon conditions: time to change a confusing terminology. Arthroscopy 1998;14(8):840–3.
30. Jarvinen TAH, Kannus P, Maffulli N, et al. Achilles tendon disorders: etiology and epidemiology. Foot Ankle Clin 2005;10(2):255–66.
31. Maffulli N, Wong J, Almekinders LC. Types and epidemiology of tendinopathy. Clin Sports Med 2003;22(4):675–92.
32. Feilmeier M. Non-insertional Achilles tendinopathy pathological background and clinical examination. Clin Podiatr Med Surg 2017;34:129–36.
33. Holmes GB, Lin J. Etiologic factors associated with symptomatic Achilles tendinopathy. Foot Ankle Int 2006;27(11):952–9.
34. Corrao G, Zambon A, Bertu L, et al. Evidence of tendonitis provoked by fluoroquinolone treatment: a case-control study. Drug Saf 2006;29(10):889–96.
35. Vora AM, Myerson MS, Oliva F, et al. Tendinopathy of the main body of the Achilles tendon. Foot Ankle Clin 2005;10(2):293–308.

36. Longo U, Ronga M, Maffulli N. Achilles tendinopathy. Sports Med Arthrosc Rev 2009;17(2):112–26.
37. Leadbetter WB. Cell-matrix response in tendon injury. Clin Sports Med 1992;11: 533–78.
38. Rufai A, Ralphs JR, Benjamin M, et al. Structure and histopathology of the insertional region of the human Achilles tendon. J Orthop Res 1995;13(4):585–93.
39. Benjamin M, Rufai A, Ralphs JR, et al. The mechanism of formation of bony spurs (enthesophytes) in the Achilles tendon. Arthritis Rheum 2000;4393:576–83.
40. Chimenti RL, Cychosz CC, Hall MM, et al. Current concepts review update: insertional Achilles tendinopathy. Foot Ankle Int 2017;38(10):1160–9.
41. Chimenti RL, Bucklin M, Kelly M, et al. Insertional Achilles tendinopathy associated with altered transverse compressive and axial tensile strain during ankle dorsiflexion. J Orthop Res 2017;35(4):910–5.
42. Gurdezi S, Kohls-Gatzoulis J, Solan MC. Results of proximal medial gastrocnemius release for Achilles tendinopathy. Foot Ankle Int 2013;34(10):1364–9.
43. Kiewiet NJ, Holthusen SM, Bohay DR, et al. Gastrocnemius recession for chronic non-insertional Achilles tendinopathy. Foot Ankle Int 2013;34(4):481–5.
44. Kaufman KR, Brodine Sk, Shaffer RA, et al. The effect of foot structure and range of motion on musculoskeletal overuse injuries. Am J Sports Med 1999;27(5): 585–93.
45. Mahieu NN, Witvrouw E, Stevens V, et al. Intrinsic risk factors for the development of Achilles tendon overuse injury: a prospective study. Am J Sports Med 2006; 34(2):226–35.
46. Maffulli N, Kenward M, Testa V, et al. Clinical diagnosis of Achilles tendinopathy with tendinosis. Clin J Sport Med 2003;13(1):11–5.
47. van Sterkenburg MN, Muller B, Maas M, et al. Appearance of the weight-bearing lateral radiograph in retrocalcaneal bursitis. Acta Orthop 2010;81(3):387–90.
48. Shibuya N, Thorud JC, Agarwal MR, et al. Is calcaneal inclination higher in patients with insertional Achilles tendinosis? A case-controlled, cross-sectional study. J Foot Ankle Surg 2021;51(6):757–61.

The Spring Ligament Complex—Anatomy and Function

Andrew M. Belis, DPM, FACFAS, FASPS*,
Gregory A. Foote, DPM, AACFAS

KEYWORDS

- Calcaneonavicular ligament • Spring ligament complex • Talonavicular joint
- Pes planovalgus • Posterior tibial tendon dysfunction • Arch collapse
- Midtarsal joint • Flatfoot

KEY POINTS

- The spring ligament complex is a combination of 3 separate ligaments making up 2 discrete bundles to provide support to the talar head and talonavicular joint.
- The superomedial portion of the ligament is the most robust and crucial of the constituents but is most prone to damage.
- This ligament complex functions in conjunction with the dynamic structures of the foot, such as the posterior tibial tendon and plantar fascia, to provide support of the medial longitudinal arch.
- Diagnosis of spring ligament rupture or insufficiency may be accomplished with clinical examination, radiographs, and MRI findings.
- Failure of the spring ligament is commonly seen in advanced stages of pes planus or more rarely in acute trauma.

INTRODUCTION: ANATOMY OF THE SPRING LIGAMENT COMPLEX

The spring ligament, or calcaneonavicular ligament (CNL), is a thick triangular band of tissue that serves as a connection between the calcaneus and the navicular to provide support to the medial longitudinal arch of the foot.[1] This unique structure has a combination of interlacing fibers and fibrocartilage to provide resistance to bending and tensile forces.[2] The spring ligament works in conjunction with the anterior and middle facets of the calcaneus as well as the talar articulation of the navicular to form the acetabulum pedis, providing support to the talar head.[3] In the original description of the spring ligament in 1896, Smith[4] paralleled the similarities of this joint complex to that of the diarthrodial hip joint, thereby coining the complex as the acetabulum pedis. In

Orthopedic Center of Florida, 12670 Creekside Lane, Suite 202, Fort Myers, FL 33919, USA
* Corresponding author.
E-mail address: Dr.Belis@ocfla.net
Twitter: @drandrewbelis (A.M.B.)

Clin Podiatr Med Surg 39 (2022) 393–403
https://doi.org/10.1016/j.cpm.2022.02.003
0891-8422/22/© 2022 Elsevier Inc. All rights reserved.

podiatric.theclinics.com

each of these articulations, a rounded head is held into a deep extensive socket, where the articular surface of the socket is primarily cartilaginous. The spring ligament complex contributes the floor and medial portion of the acetabulum pedis and is composed of 2 major constituents: the superomedial CNL and the inferior CNL, separated by a triangle-shaped area of fatty tissue.[2] Further descriptions have described the inferior portion as a combination of 2 separate ligaments, the medioplantar oblique CNL and the inferoplantar longitudinal CNL owing to a difference in orientation of ligamentous fibers between these structures.[5,6]

Superomedial Calcaneonavicular Ligament

The superomedial CNL is the primary contributor of the spring ligament complex. This is the strongest and broadest of the 3 structures, measuring between 2 and 4 mm in thickness.[6,7] These ligamentous fibers originate from the sustentaculum tali and anterior facet of the calcaneus, where they combine with the attachment of the tibiocalcaneal fibers of the superficial deltoid ligament. The fibers are oriented in a curved medial to lateral direction on the superomedial aspect of the sustentaculum tali and follow the contour of the medial aspect of the anterior calcaneal facet.[2] Coursing distally, the plantar aspect of this structure expands to accommodate the posterior tibial tendon (PTT) sheath, where a flattened area exists, corresponding to the path of the PTT. This ligament ultimately progresses to insert at the inferior and superomedial aspect of the navicular (**Fig. 1**).

The insertion point of the superomedial CNL completely lines the superior, medial, and inferior portion of the medial articular surface of the navicular. Here, the ligament shares the insertion of the PTT; however, this does not directly insert into the tuberosity.[2] The deep, central, articular portion of the superomedial bundle is covered by fibrocartilage to facilitate interaction with the talar head.[7] This area resembles a triangular articular facet that corresponds to the plantar-medial triangular facet of the talar head itself (**Fig. 2**).[2] This aspect of the ligament is separated from the PTT insertion by a "gliding zone" that is lined with a single layer of synovial cells.[5]

Inferior Calcaneonavicular Ligament

The inferior CNL has been classically described as a separate structure to the superomedial portion of the ligament that is inferior and plantar, corresponding to the lower aspect of the talar head. Further cadaveric studies have revealed that this is actually a combination of 2 distinctly separate structures, the medioplantar oblique CNL and the inferoplantar longitudinal CNL (see **Figs. 1** and **2**; **Fig. 3**).[5]

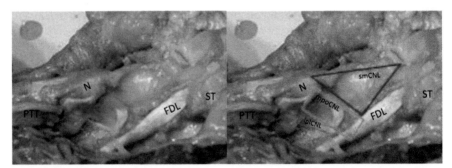

Fig. 1. Medial view of the spring ligament complex. FDL, flexor digitorum longus tendon; iplCNL, inferoplantar longitudinal calcaneonavicular ligament (*orange*); mpoCNL, medioplantar oblique calcaneonavicular ligament (*green*); N, navicular; smCNL, superomedial calcaneonavicular ligament (*red*); ST, sustentaculum tali.

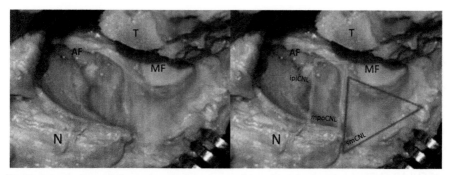

Fig. 2. Dorsal view of the spring ligament complex with talar head removed. AF, anterior calcaneal facet; MF, middle calcaneal facet; T, talus (talar head removed).

Medioplantar oblique calcaneonavicular ligament
The medioplantar oblique CNL is a trapezoidal-shaped ligament, measuring less than 4 mm in thickness, located between the superomedial CNL and the inferoplantar CNL.[5,6,8] The structure begins at the coronoid fossa, a small fossa that is anterior to the middle calcaneal facet at the anterior portion of the calcaneus (see **Fig. 3**). This then courses in an oblique orientation to insert below the navicular tuberosity at the medial and plantar portion of the navicular bone.[9] MRI evaluation has revealed this as a distinct ligament because of its course, insertion, and laminated appearance.[5]

Inferoplantar longitudinal calcaneonavicular ligament
The second of these structures, the inferoplantar longitudinal CNL, is a short, thick, quadrilateral-shaped ligament, measuring less than 4 mm in thickness, located at the most lateral portion of the spring ligament complex.[8,10] The inferoplantar longitudinal CNL originates at the coronoid fossa just anterior to the medioplantar oblique CNL, where it is separated by a fat layer. This extends distally, nearly parallel to the long axis of the foot, to a distinct insertion at the inferior beak of the midnavicular, just lateral to that of the superomedial CNL (see **Figs. 2** and **3**).[2,5] This completes the lateral and plantar portion of the spring ligament complex, giving its resemblance to a socket.

Spring ligament recess
A potential space exists between the medial plantar oblique and the inferoplantar longitudinal bands that is referred to as the spring ligament recess. This is an important

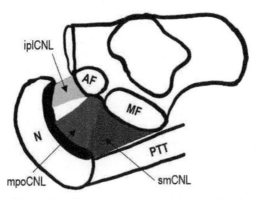

Fig. 3. Dorsal view of the spring ligament complex with the talus absent.

anatomic characteristic, as this may be falsely implicated as a spring ligament tear on MRI. This space has a direct connection with the talonavicular joint (TNJ) and is lined by synovium adjacent to both the talonavicular and the subtalar joint. This should be differentiated from a spring ligament tear by the presence of discrete borders and a homogeneous fluid signal in an interval between the medial plantar oblique and the inferoplantar longitudinal portions of the ligament complex.[11] This space can also be directly visualized by performing an arthrogram of the TNJ. With this technique, contrast is visualized, accumulating in the space immediately inferior to the TNJ (**Fig. 4**). Evaluation of this structure should be considered with scrutiny in the radiological diagnosis of an acute ligament tear.

VASCULAR SUPPLY

The spring ligament obtains its primary vascular supply from its proximal and distal bony attachments from calcaneus and navicular, respectively. The calcaneal branches of the medial plantar artery supply the proximal one-third to one-half of the ligament via direct penetration and through its bony origin at the sustentaculum tali.[2] The navicular branches of the medial plantar artery and the bony attachments to the navicular provide the major supply to the distal one-third to one-half of the ligament. This leaves a central area of avascular tissue (**Fig. 5**), including the dorsal one-third that lacks adequate perfusion and therefore is predisposed to injury.[2]

FUNCTION

The term spring ligament has been frequently described but may be a misnomer owing to the absence of elastin or elastic fibers within the CNL in histologic studies. The ligamentous tissue is composed of densely packed collagen bundles and has no inherent elastic properties.[2,12] This structure instead acts as more of a sling rather than a spring, whereby the interlacing fibers of the complex form a gentle concavity around the talar head.[2] Primarily, the function of the CNL as a whole is to provide stability to the TNJ.[13] In addition, the interaction with the deltoid ligament, plantar fascia, and the

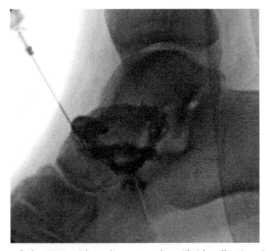

Fig. 4. Arthrogram of the TNJ with radiopaque dye. Fluid collection is visualized at the plantar aspect of the talar head representing the spring ligament recess.

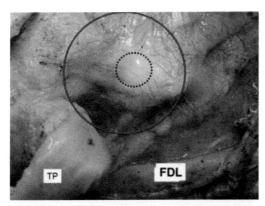

Fig. 5. Chinese ink infiltrated to local blood supply of the spring ligament. (*circle*) Area of perfusion with inner circle depicting avascular zone. TP, posterior tibial tendon. (Reprinted with permission from Vadell AM, Peratta A. Calcaneonavicular Ligament. Foot and Ankle Clinics, 2012; 17(3): 437-448.[14])

PTT contributes to stability of the subtalar and ankle joint.[14] This makes the spring ligament a major anatomic contributor to the integrity of the medial longitudinal arch, forming the floor for the course of the PTT on 1 side and a sling for the talar head on the other.[2,15] The dorsal fibrocartilaginous surface of the superomedial CNL aids in its resistance to compression and stress at the TNJ.[14] The histology and microvascular studies reveal this portion of the ligament to be essentially avascular, much like the meniscus of the knee (**Fig. 6**).[16]

This region is lined by synovial cells and contains loose connective tissue to additionally offer a smooth surface for articulation throughout ambulation.[5] The superomedial CNL is intimately interlaced with the superficial deltoid ligament, thereby providing additional resistance to the medial compressive forces of the hindfoot.[9,17,18] The biomechanical analysis of this complex shows that the superomedial CNL is the strongest of the ligaments in the complex. The inferior portion of the ligament, conversely, has been shown to have a minimal biomechanical role in stabilization at the TNJ and longitudinal arch of the foot.[2] This suggests that the superomedial and inferior CNL are part of the group of ligaments that support the medial longitudinal arch, but could not hold up the arch alone.

FAILURE PRESENTATION

The vast majority of spring ligament failure is seen in those with long-standing pes planus deformity and subsequent failure of support to the medial longitudinal arch. Acute injuries to the spring ligament do occur; however, these are exceedingly rare and typically result from an explosive mechanism or severe pronation trauma that can lead to dislocation at the TNJ.[18–22] The sequela of this injury involves a loss of integrity of the medial longitudinal arch leading to eventual collapse and may, in turn, lead to an acquired flatfoot deformity. A damaged spring ligament complex must be repaired in these injuries, as this structure is an essential anatomic constituent to the integrity of the medial arch, especially in cases whereby the dynamic support of the PTT has been compromised.[15]

Failure of the spring ligament complex is most frequently encountered with dysfunction of the PTT. The disruption of this ligament must be considered when evaluating those with PTT dysfunction, as the clinical symptoms may mimic and coincide with

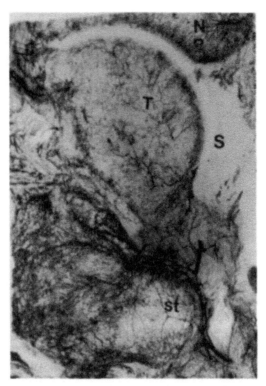

Fig. 6. Transverse section of spring ligament complex with modified Spalteholz technique to visualize microvascular supply revealing central area of avascular tissue (*white*). S, superomedial calcaneonavicular ligament; st, sustentaculum tali. T, Talus; N, Navicular. (*From* Davis WH, Sobel M, DiCarlo EF, Torzilli PA, Deng X, Geppert MJ, Patel MB, Deland J. Gross, histological, and microvascular anatomy and biomechanical testing of the spring ligament complex. Foot Ankle Int. 1996 Feb;17(2):95-102. https://doi.org/10.1177/107110079601700207. PMID: 8919408.)

the advanced stages of acquired flatfoot deformity. The superomedial band is most commonly involved in spring ligament tears followed by the medioplantar oblique band.[23,24] In PTT dysfunction, the repetitive plantarflexory force of the talar head into the spring ligament complex results in attenuation and eventual tearing. This progresses to a further plantarflexion of the talus, forefoot abduction, and hindfoot valgus deformity.[8]

Advanced imaging techniques, such as MRI, may be helpful in the diagnosis of a spring ligament tear; however, because of the complexity in orientation of the multiple fibrous bands, this modality may provide inconsistent findings. In addition, the proximity to the PTT poses implications for inaccurate diagnosis of a discrete ligamentous rupture or insufficiency, as these pathologic conditions will typically coincide. One study by Yao et al in 1999 showed that the sensitivity of MRI for the diagnosis of spring ligament damage ranges from 54% to 77%, whereas the specificity was 100%.[25] In regard to specific MRI findings, acute ruptures manifest as high signal intensity on T2-weighted or long time to echo (TE) images. Chronic ligamentous tears, in contrast, are less likely to exhibit hypersensitivity on T2-weighted images. Spring ligament signal changes on MRI were more frequently observed in patients with PTT dysfunction than those with a healthy PTT, as is to be expected with the close relationship among these conditions.[13,25].Most MRI studies of symptomatic flatfeet will show concomitant abnormality in the spring ligament when damage is noted in the PTT.

Clinically, patients with spring ligament injuries present with pain and tenderness to the medial aspect of the arch, between the talar head and navicular tuberosity. This may be accompanied by swelling, erythema, plantar medial callosity, and in severe cases, talar head protrusion. As the superomedial portion of the spring ligament complex is torn, the talar head is allowed to escape from its confinement within the navicular, where it begins to plantarflex leading to subsequent abduction of the forefoot (**Fig. 7**).

Patients with spring ligament insufficiency will present in a similar fashion to those with advanced PTT dysfunction. As the talus advances to a more vertical position, there will be a resultant drop of the medial longitudinal arch and pain related to difficulty in single-limb support.[5]

Maintenance of the medial longitudinal arch and midfoot stability relies on both dynamic and static stabilization. The major dynamic stabilizer of the hindfoot and ankle is the PTT, whereas static stabilization of the medial longitudinal arch is provided by the spring ligament and plantar fascia. Therefore, in cases whereby the PTT fails or becomes insufficient, excess stress is transferred to these static ligamentous stabilizers of the arch. When pronatory stress progresses through the medial longitudinal arch and is transferred to the deltoid ligament, the main static stabilizer at the ankle, this leads to findings of a stage 4 flatfoot deformity and tibiotalar subluxation.

On clinical weight-bearing examination, a decrease in medial longitudinal arch height with talar head collapse is also suggestive of spring ligament insufficiency. These patients may present with a milder forefoot abduction and neutral hindfoot position with loss of arch integrity (**Fig. 8**).

Isolated spring ligament insufficiency may present with a different clinical appearance in the presence of a diseased versus healthy PTT. In isolated ligament tears or insufficiency without PTT dysfunction, the rearfoot weight-bearing examination shows the typical "too many toes" sign and everted calcaneus; however, the dynamic heel rise test may fail to completely invert heel and correct abduction. This clinical finding of only a partial deformity reversal may be a more definitive predictor for isolated spring ligament insufficiency.[26] When spring ligament deficiency presents in conjunction with PTT dysfunction, a complete absence of heel inversion and persistent forefoot abduction are apparent with the dynamic heel rise test.

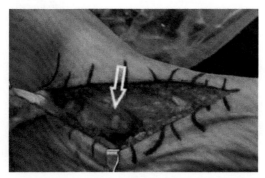

Fig. 7. Spring ligament tear with protrusion of talar head. (*Arrow*) Site of tear at the superomedial CNL with PTT and FDL tendon reflected.

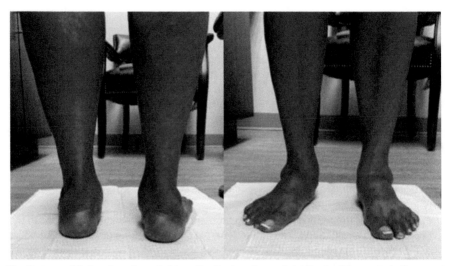

Fig. 8. Loss of integrity of medial longitudinal arch on right foot with neutral alignment maintained to the left foot.

The neutral heel lateral push test is another reliable clinical examination test to determine the integrity of the spring ligament complex separately from the integrity of the PTT. This is performed while holding the calcaneus in neutral position with 1 hand while stressing the TNJ with a medial force applied to the first ray. Resistance felt with stress in abduction of the TNJ indicates an intact spring ligament, whereas

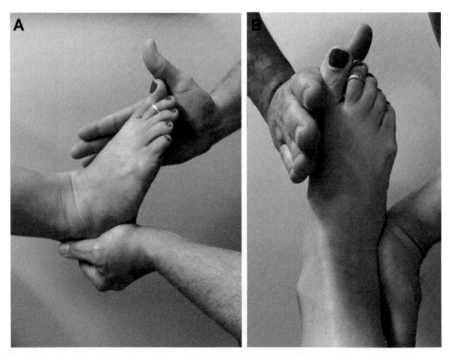

Fig. 9. Neutral heel lateral push test. (*A*) Lateral foot view. (*B*) Dorsal foot view push test.

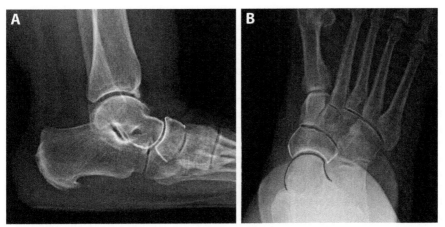

Fig. 10. (*A*) Weight-bearing lateral radiograph with talonavicular fault and increase in talar declination angle. (*B*) Weight-bearing anteroposterior radiograph with talar head uncovering and increase in Kite angle.

unrestricted abduction movement indicates loss of integrity of the spring ligament. A study of this maneuver by Pasapula and colleagues[27] provides support that isolated spring ligament failure plays a more important role in the development of pes plano-valgus than PPT dysfunction alone (**Fig. 9**).

Previous radiographic studies have also evaluated the impact of either PTT insufficiency or ligament support on the development of the flatfoot deformity. By evaluation of an in vitro model, Deland and colleagues[28] found that the clinical and radiographic deformity associated with chronic PTT insufficiency was not observed in isolated release of the PTT. Instead, they concluded that the radiographic deformity occurred only when concurrent spring ligament damage was present. Radiographic findings are most readily visible on the weight-bearing lateral view, where a talonavicular fault or incongruity exists at the TNJ. This is more clearly defined by a subsequent and gradual increase in talar declination angle and loss of calcaneal pitch. The weight-bearing anteroposterior view is also valuable in the diagnosis of spring ligament insufficiency with talar head uncovering medially and a significant increase in Kite angle (**Fig. 10**).

Clinical and radiographic findings provide crucial information in the diagnosis of spring ligament insufficiency. These findings must be used for an accurate and effective evaluation of the specific structures that contribute to the acquired flatfoot deformity. Furthermore, these findings and studies provide further evidence of how crucial the reconstruction of the spring ligament complex is when repairing the dynamic support structures of the medial longitudinal arch.

SUMMARY

Understanding the anatomy of the ligamentous components of the talo-calcaneal-navicular joint is essential to fully appreciate this complex support system for the arch and its function in normal gait. Although classically described as the spring ligament, this term may be somewhat misleading. Primarily, this is due to the notion that this was 1 ligament; however, anatomically, this has been proven to be a combination of 3 separately distinct structures. Although the superomedial CNL is the strongest and broadest of these structures, it is most susceptible to injury owing to its location and its avascular nature. In addition, this ligament may also be prone to attenuation rather than a complete tear, especially if the structures that help support the arch more gradually begin to fail. The fibrocartilaginous content of the ligament indicates that this is exposed to repetitive tension while also allowing for a gliding motion of the talar head with compression from the adjacent PTT. Second, and of equal importance, the function of the spring ligament is not that of a spring but more that of a sling for static support for the arch.

The integrity of the medial longitudinal arch relies on the support of both the static (ligamentous) and dynamic (tendinous) stabilizers of the foot. The use of advanced imaging techniques in conjunction with radiographic and clinical findings provide the practitioner with a more accurate diagnosis of spring ligament insufficiency and its relationship to the surrounding structures and its impact on arch support. The spring ligament complex provides vital anatomic support of the medial longitudinal arch and must be appropriately addressed when damaged or insufficient. This is especially important in those presenting with a deficiency of the PTT, or when the dynamic support of the medial longitudinal arch has been compromised. This is due not only to the inherent support this structure offers to the acetabulum pedis but also the entirety of the medial collateral complex of the ankle joint and hindfoot. Failure to recognize a spring ligament injury as a cause of the flatfoot deformity could ultimately lead to inappropriate operative management and unsatisfactory patient outcomes.

CLINICS CARE POINTS

- This article presents a detailed explanation of the anatomy and function of the spring ligament.
- There is a positive correlation between the integrity of the spring ligament and the stability of the arch.

DISCLOSURE

The authors have nothing to disclose.

REFERENCES

1. Melão L, Canella C, Weber M, et al. Ligaments of the transverse tarsal joint complex: MRI anatomic correlation in cadavers. Am J Roentgenol 2009;193:662–71.
2. Davis WH, Sobel M, DiCarlo EF, et al. Histological, and microvascular anatomy and biomechanical testing of the spring ligament complex. Foot Ankle Int 1996;17:95–102.
3. Nazarenko A, Beltran LS, Bencardino JT. Imaging evaluation of traumatic ligamentous injuries of the ankle and foot. Radiol Clin North Am 2013;51:455–78.
4. Smith EB. The astragalo-calcaneo-navicular joint. J Anat Physiol 1986;30(238): 290–412.
5. Mengiardi B, Zanetti M, Schottle P, et al. Spring ligament complex: MR imaging-anatomic correlation and findings in asymptomatic subjects. Radiology 2005; 237(1):242–9.
6. Taniguchi A, Tanaka Y, Takakura Y, et al. Anatomy of the spring ligament. J Bone Joint Surg Am 2003;85-A:2174–8.
7. Patil V, Ebraheim NA, Frogameni A, et al. Morphometric dimensions of the calcaneonavicular (spring) ligament. Foot Ankle Int 2007;28:927–32.

8. Omar H, Saini V, Wadhwa V, et al. Spring ligament complex: illustrated normal anatomy and spectrum of pathologies on 3T MR imaging. Eur J Radiol 2016; 85(11):2133–43.
9. Sarrafian SK. Anatomy of the foot and ankle: descriptive, topographic, functional. Philadelphia: Lippincott; 1983. p. 159–282.
10. Ngai SS, Tafur M, Chang EY, et al. Magnetic resonance imaging of ankle ligaments. Can Assoc Radiol J 2016;67:60–8.
11. Desai KR, Beltran LS, Bencardino JT, et al. The spring ligament recess of the talocalcaneonavicular joint: depiction on MR images with cadaveric and histologic correlation. Am J Roentgenol 2011;196:1145–50.
12. Hardy RH. Observations on the structure and properties of the plantar calcaneonavicular ligament in man. J Anat 1951;85:135–9.
13. Rule J, Yao L, Seeger LL. Spring ligament of the ankle: normal MR anatomy. Am J Roentgenol 1993;161:1241–4.
14. Vadell AM, Peratta A. Calcaneonavicular ligament. Foot Ankle Clin 2012;17(3): 437–48.
15. Gazdag AR, Cracchiolo A 3rd. Rupture of the posterior tibial tendon. Evaluation of injury of the spring ligament and clinical assessment of tendon transfer and ligament repair. J Bone Joint Surg Am 1997;79:675–81.
16. Arnoczky SP, Warren RF. Microvasculature of the human meniscus. Am J Sports Med 1982;10:90–5.
17. Hamilton WG. Surgical anatomy of the foot and ankle. Ciba Clin Symp 1985; 37(3):4.
18. Toye LR, Helms CA, Hoffman BD, et al. MRI of spring ligament tears. Am J Roentgenol 2005;184:1475–80.
19. Borton DC, Saxby TS. Tear of the plantar calcaneonavicular (spring) ligament causing flatfoot. A case report. J Bone Joint Surg Br 1997;79:641–3.
20. Orr JD, Nunley JA 2nd. Isolated spring ligament failure as a cause of adult-acquired flatfoot deformity. Foot Ankle Int 2013;34:818–23.
21. Subhas N, Sundaram M. Diagnosis: isolated spring ligament tear demonstrated on magnetic resonance imaging. Orthopedics 2007;30(1):70–2.
22. Chen JP, Allen AM. MR diagnosis of traumatic tear of the spring ligament in a pole vaulter. Skeletal Radiol 1997;26:310–2.
23. Jahss MH. Spontaneous rupture of the tibialis posterior tendon: clinical findings, tenographic studies, and a new technique of repair. Foot Ankle 1982;3:158–66.
24. Sarrafian SK. Anatomy of the foot and ankle. Philadelphia: J.B. Lippincott; 1983. p. 157–75.
25. Yao L, Gentili A, Cracchiolo A. MR imaging findings in spring ligament insufficiency. Skeletal Radiol May 1999;28(5):245–50.
26. Masaragian HJ, Massetti S, Fernando DP, et al. Flatfoot deformity due to isolated spring ligament injury. J Foot Ankle Surg 2020;59(3):469–78.
27. Pasapula C, Devany A, Magan A, et al. Neutral heel lateral push test: the first clinical examination of spring ligament integrity. The Foot 2015;25(2):69–74.
28. Deland JT, Arnoczky SP, Thompson FM. Adult acquired flatfoot deformity at the talonavicular joint: reconstruction of the spring ligament in an in vitro model. Foot & Ankle 1992;13(6):327–32.

Gross Anatomy
Achilles Tendon

Jason Kayce, DPM, FACFAS

KEYWORDS

- Achilles • Anatomy • Tendon • Gross

KEY POINTS

- Gross overview of the anatomic composition of the Achilles tendon.
- A review of the relationship of the gastrocnemius, soleus, and plantaris in the formation of the Achilles tendon.
- In depth evaluation of the vascularity and nerve supply of the Achilles tendon.

INTRODUCTION

The Achilles tendon is the strongest tendon in the body. It is composed of the gastrocnemius and soleus muscles, and often the plantaris muscle.[1,2] The muscles and the Achilles tendon are located within the posterior, superficial compartment of the calf. The Achilles is the main plantar flexor of the ankle.[3,4]

GASTROCNEMIUS

The medial and lateral heads of the gastrocnemius originate proximal to the knee from the femoral condyles. The medial head of the gastrocnemius arises from the popliteal surface of the femur behind the medial supracondylar line and adductor tubercle, above the medial femoral condyle. The medial head of the gastrocnemius is larger and longer than the lateral head.[4]

The lateral head of the gastrocnemius is shorter and arises from the posterior aspect of the lateral femoral condyle, above and posterior to the lateral epicondyle, as well as from a portion of the lateral lip of the linea aspera superior to the lateral condyle. Both the medial and the lateral heads also originate from the oblique popliteal ligament, a portion of the knee joint capsule, and are attached to the condyles of the femur by strong flat tendons, which extend for a short distance on the posterior or the superficial surface of these muscles as an aponeurosis.[2]

Bursae may lie deep to the medial and lateral heads of the gastrocnemius. The bursa deep to the medial head can communicate with the knee joint and may be

Midwestern University Arizona College of Podiatric Medicine, Paradise Valley Foot & Ankle, 4611 East Shea Boulevard, Phoenix, AZ 85028, USA
E-mail address: jasonkayce@gmail.com

Clin Podiatr Med Surg 39 (2022) 405–410
https://doi.org/10.1016/j.cpm.2022.03.003
0891-8422/22/© 2022 Elsevier Inc. All rights reserved.

involved in Baker cysts. The deep surface of the gastrocnemius is tendinous. The muscle belly of the gastrocnemius extends to the middle of the calf. As the medial and lateral muscle bellies conjoin, they form a tenderness raphe that becomes continuous with the aponeurosis about the anterior or deep aspect of the muscle. This aponeurosis unites with the tendon of the soleus to form the Achilles tendon.[2]

SOLEUS

The soleus muscle is a broad, flat pennate muscle. The soleus is wider than the gastrocnemius, and its muscle fibers extend more distally than the gastrocnemius. The soleus originates from the posterior surface of the head and upper fourth of the posterior surface of the fibula, from a fibrils arch between the fibula and tibia, and from the oblique line and the middle third of the medial border of the tibia.[2] The popliteal vessels and the tibial nerve pass under the fibrils arch. The soleus muscle consists of 2 aponeurotic lamellae with the bulk of the vascular multipennate muscle fibers in between. The muscular fibers end in the posterior aponeurosis of the soleus, which lies anterior to the aponeurosis of the gastrocnemius. The aponeurotic fibers of the muscles lie parallel to each other before they unite.[5] The soleus fuses with the gastrocnemius and forms the deepest portion of the Achilles tendon.

The tendinous component of the soleus is the largest of the tendons that comprise the Achilles tendon. It is the prime plantar flexor.[6,7] The soleus is a postural muscle that keeps the body vertical during stance. Although the gastrocnemius also has an effect on the knee joint, the soleus only acts upon the ankle joint. As the center of gravity passes in front of the axis of movement of the knee joint, the soleus contracts to counteract the tendency for the body to tilt forward at the ankle.[8]

The soleus may consist of 2 anomalies that are recognized. The first is an extension of the muscle more distally than usual along the Achilles tendon. The second is a separate insertion of the soleus into the superior surface of the calcaneus with a separate tendon or directly without a tendon.[2]

PLANTARIS

The plantaris muscle has a variable size and is absent in 6% to 8% of the population. The plantaris has a short, fleshy origin from the popliteal surface of the femur above the lateral aspect of the femoral condyle. The muscle belly is typically 5 to 10 cm in length followed by a long tendon that extends distally between the gastrocnemius and soleus. The plantaris tendon inserts into the medial border of the Achilles tendon, anterior to the Achilles tendon.[2] In 6% to 8% of individuals, it inserts into the flexor retinaculum.[5] This tendon is often commonly sacrificed as a tendon graft during surgical procedures where donor tendon is required.

ACHILLES TENDON

In total, the Achilles tendon is approximately 15 cm long. The Achilles tendon originates at the myotendinous junction of the gastrocnemius and soleus in the middle of the calf. The Achilles tendon fully incorporates approximately 8 cm to set to 10 cm above the calcaneal insertion site.[1] The Achilles tendon transitioned proximally to distally from flat to rounded to flat. The Achilles tendon is flattened from the myotendinous junction and becomes rounded approximately 4 cm from its insertion into the calcaneus. At the insertion level, the tendon flattens and expands, becoming cartilaginous to insert onto a rough area on the middle of the lower aspect of the posterior surface of the calcaneus. On the anterior surface of the tendon, it receives the muscular fibers from the soleus almost to the level of its insertion.[9,10] The anterior and medial aspects of the tendon receive fibers from the soleus, and the posterior aspect is derived from gastrocnemius fibers.[11] These contributions and proportions from the gastrocnemius and soleus vary among individuals.

As the Achilles tendon descends, it rotates 90° such that gastrocnemius fibers attach laterally and posteriorly while fibers of the soleus attach medially and anteriorly.[12] The rotation of tendinous fibers originates above the region where the soleus tends to join the gastrocnemius. The degree of rotation is greater if there is minimal fusion of the gastrocnemius and soleus components. This spiraling has been shown to result in less fiber buckling when the tendon is lax and less deformation when tension is applied to the tendon.[12] This twisting of the Achilles as it descends was thought to produce an area of stress within the tendon, which is most notable 2 cm to 5 cm proximal to its calcaneal insertion.[13,14] This has been further evaluated and has led to controversy regarding the reality of a "watershed" region of the Achilles tendon.

The Achilles tendon insertion broadens distally and has a wide deltoid type of attachment, which varies from 1.2 cm to 2.5 cm.[15] The deep surface of the inferior portion of the tendon above its attachment to the calcaneus has an area of fibrocartilage between the tendon and the superior aspect of the calcaneus, where there is a similar area of fibrocartilage.[13,16] Deep and immediately proximal to the Achilles insertion is the retrocalcaneal bursa, which is interpositioned between the tendon and the posterior calcaneal tuberosity.[11]

Some of the collagen fibers at the insertion of the Achilles tendon form Sharpey fibers and become continuous with fibrils tissue overlying the calcaneus. The endotenon becomes continuous with the periosteum. There is no periosteum at the Achilles insertion.[6,7] Some of the superficial fibers may become continuous with fibrils tissue of the calcaneus and pass from the lower border of the calcaneus to join the plantar fascia.[16,17] The number of fibers that connect the Achilles tendon to the plantar fascia decrease with age.[2]

The Achilles tendon is enclosed by a paratenon, which serves as an elastic sleeve to allow gliding. There is no true synovial sheath surrounding the Achilles tendon. This paratenon is a thin gliding membrane of loose areolar tissue that is rich in mucopolysaccharides. It is composed of sheets of dense connective tissue that separate the tendon from the deep fascia of the leg. The peritendinous structure and the abundance of mucopolysaccharides within the sheath allow sliding of the tendon along adjacent tissues. The proximal aspect of the paratenon is continuous with the muscle fascia, and distally, it blends with the periosteum of the calcaneus.[11]

HISTOLOGY OF THE ACHILLES TENDON

The Achilles tendon is composed of parallel bundles of type 1 collagen.[1] The average size of the collagen fibers of the Achilles tendon is 60 μm. These collagen fibers are organized into fibrils, which vary from 30 nm to 130 nm in diameter, yet most are between 50 and 90 nm in diameter.[2] A group of fibers is organized into fascicles, which are further grouped into bundles. Individual fibrils do not course the entire length of the tendon, but rather are linked in succession, requiring transfer of stress between associated fibril units.[1] Within the midsubstance of the tendon are fibroblasts that are arranged in longitudinal rows.[11] Around each collagen bundle is an endotenon, which maintains the bundle's integrity. The endotenon contains vessels, lymphatics, and nerves. Surrounding the entire gross Achilles tendon lays a connective tissue sheath called the epitenon with mesotenon and paratenon on overlying it.[11]

BLOOD SUPPLY

The blood supply of tendons is variable. The blood supply about the Achilles tendon is typically divided into 3 regions: the myotendinous junction, direct supply to the tendon, and the tendon-bone interface. Blood vessels originate from vessels in the perimysium, in the periosteum, and by way of the paratenon and mesotenon. The main blood supply to the midsubstance of the Achilles tendon extends from the paratenon. The small blood vessels in the paratenon course transversely toward the tendon and branch several times before coursing parallel to the long access of the tendon. The vessels enter the Achilles tendon along the endotenon. The recurrent branch of the posterior tibial artery supplies the proximal aspect of the tendon while the distal tendon is supplied by the rete arteriosum calcaneare and by the fibular and posterior tibial arteries. Vessels that supply the bone tendon interface supply the lower third of the tendon. There are indirect anastomoses between vessels supplying the midsubstance of the tendon and vessels at the bone tendon interface.[2]

NERVE SUPPLY

Tendons are supplied by sensory nerves from the overlying superficial nerves or from nearby deep nerves, the tibial nerve, and its branches number.[9] The nerve supply is largely afferent. Afferent receptors are found near the myotendinous junction.[9] These may be found either on the surface of the tendon or in the tendon. The nerves form a longitudinal plexus and enter by way of the septa of the endotenon or the mesotenon if there is a synovial sheath. Branches may also pass from the paratenon via the epitenon to reach the surface or the interior of a tendon.[18,19]

BIOMECHANICS

The Achilles tendon is subjected to the highest loads in the body. It can withstand tensile loads up to 12 times body weight. The gastrocnemius and soleus muscles combine to form the main plantar flexors of the foot at the level of the ankle. Because it crosses the knee joint, the gastrocnemius is also a contributor to knee flexion. Silver and colleagues[20] suggested that the soleus is the main plantar flexor at the ankle during normal gait. They showed the soleus to exert nearly double the plantar flexion force at the ankle compared with the gastrocnemius.[20]

The size and unique characteristics of the Achilles tendon allow it to function under high stress. This ability to function under high stress creates potential for repetitive stress injury. The stress-strain resistance properties of the Achilles are similar to all tendons, with physiologic collagen fiber stretching occurring from 2% to 4% stretch length, microscopic fibril failure at 6% to 8% stretch, and macroscopic failure beyond 8% stretch.[21] A variety of abnormalities, deformities, and activities can place loads on the Achilles tendon that are beyond its capacity to rebound, which can result in internal tendon fiber damage and degeneration. On the other hand, mechanical stress is also necessary to prevent and to recover from injury, as subrupture forces signal fibroblasts to produce collagen to aid in tendon health.[22]

WATERSHED CONTROVERSY

As previously discussed, the Achilles tendon rotates 90° as it courses from proximal to distal. In 1946, it was hypothesized that the twisting or rotating of the fibers is a possible cause of the purported ischemia of the midsubstance of the tendon.[23] This "wringing out" of the tendon has been described and observed by many. It has been thought that this area of rotation also produces an area of stress within the tendon, which is most notable 2 to 5 cm proximal to its calcaneal insertion.[12,14] However, the effect of this fiber rotation on real-time blood flow has not been proven through experimentation. Multiple studies have demonstrated uniform blood flow throughout the tendon at rest, with contracture, and with exercise.[11]

In the 1950s, cadaveric anatomic research was performed, which led to the identification of a "watershed" area.[24] Cadaveric injection and analysis of the Achilles peritendinous vessels led to the proposal of a "watershed" region. This region was further proposed as the cause of an ischemic zone and a source of weakness and rupture. It is known that the Achilles tendon receives its blood supply from 3 main sources: the myotendinous junction, direct supply to the tendon, and the tendon-bone interface. In other words, the tendon receives blood flow proximally, distally, and from peritendinous structures. Does this distribution of vessels truly lead to an area of ischemia? In 1958, Hastad and colleagues[25] tested the hemodynamic flow throughout the tendon, challenging the watershed theory. This study displayed uniform blood flow throughout the tendon. In 1994, Aström and Westlin[26] used laser Doppler flow analysis to evaluate real-time tendon circulation at rest and during contracture. Their results show blood flow evenly distributed throughout the tendon, with only a slight decrease at its insertion into the calcaneus. Other studies have shown an increase in blood flow within the tendon during exercise activity.[11]

The relationship between a potential area of stress or ischemia secondary to fiber rotation along with early cadaveric studies led to the notion of a "watershed" within the Achilles tendon. This notion has been widely accepted for years, yet it seems more correlative rather than scientifically proven. The hemodynamic component of this theory continues to be challenged. This notion of a "watershed" region seems to be more convenient as opposed to a scientific fact. Further research is necessary to analyze real-time blood flow of the tendon, and even more research is needed to identify the reason most ruptures occur 2 to 5 cm proximal to the Achilles insertion into the calcaneus.

FINANCIAL DISCLOSURE

The author has nothing to disclose.

REFERENCES

1. Benjamin M, Theobald P, Suzuki D, et al. The anatomy of the Achilles tendon. In: Maffulli N, Almekinders L, editors. The Achilles tendon. . London: Springer-Verlag; 2007. p. 5–16.
2. O'Brien M. The anatomy of the Achilles tendon. Foot Ankle Clin 2005;10(2): 225–38.
3. Williams PC, Warwick R, Dyson M, et al, editors. Gray's anatomy. 37th edition. London; 1993.
4. Warwick R, Williams PC. Gray's anatomy. 35th edition. Edinburgh (Scotland): Longmans; 1973.
5. Hollinshead WH. Anatomy for surgeons. 2nd edition. The back and limbs, 3. Harper and Row Publishers; 1969.
6. Kvist M. Achilles tendon overuse injuries [doctoral dissertation]. Turku (Finalnd): University of Turku; 1991.
7. Kvist M. Achilles tendon injuries in athletes. Sports Med 1994;18:173–201.
8. Plastanga NP, Field D, Soames R. Anatomy and human movement structure and function. 2nd edition 1994.

9. O'Brien M. Functional anatomy and physiology of tendons. Clin Sports Med 1992; 11(3):505–20.
10. Curwin S, Tendonitis WD Standish. Its etiology and treatment. Lexington (MA): Collamore Press; 1984.
11. Dayton P. Anatomic, vascular, and mechanical overview of the Achilles tendon. Clin Podiatr Med Surg 2017;34(2):107–13.
12. Ahmed IM, Lagopoulos M, McConnell P, et al. Blood supply of the Achilles tendon. J Orthop Res 1998;16:591–6.
13. Barfred T. Experimental rupture of Achilles tendon. Acta Orthop Scand 1971;42: 528–43.
14. Benjamin M, Evans EJ, Copp L. The histology of tendon attachment to bone in man. J Anat 1986;149:89–100.
15. Schepsis AA. Achilles tendon disorders in athletes. Am J Sports Med 2002;30(2): 287–305.
16. F. Wood Jones. Structure and function as seen in the foot. Baillere, Tindall and Cox (1944).
17. Allenmark C. Partial Achilles tendon tears. Clin Sports Med 1992;11(4):759–69.
18. Jozsa G, Kannus P. Human tendons anatomy and physiology. Human Kinetics; 1997.
19. Ippolito E, Postacchini F. Anatomy. In: Perugia L, Postacchini F, Ippolito E, editors. The tendons: biology-pathology-clinical aspects. Milano (Italy): Editrice Kurtis; 1986. p. 9–36.
20. Silver RL, de la Garza J, Rang M. The myth of muscle balance. A study of relative strengths and excursions of normal muscles about the foot and ankle. J Bone Joint Surg Br 1985;67(3):432–7.
21. Wang JH. Mechanobiology of tendon. J Biomech 2006;39(9):1563–82.
22. Eliasson P, Andersson T, Hammerman M, et al. Primary gene response to mechanical loading in healing rat Achilles tendons. J Appl Physiol (1985) 2013; 114(11):1519–26.
23. Cummins EJ, Anson BJ. The structure of the calcaneal tendon (of Achilles) in relation to orthopedic surgery, with additional observations on the plantaris muscle. Surg Gynecol Obstet 1946;83:107–16.
24. Lagergren C, Lindbom A, Soderberg G. Hypervascularization in chronic inflammation demonstrated by angiography; angiographic, histopathologic, and micro-angiographic studies. Acta Radiol 1958;49(6):441–52.
25. Hastad K, Larson L, Lindholm A. Clearance of radiosodium after local deposit in the Achilles tendon. Acta Chir Scand 1958;116:251–5.
26. Aström M, Westlin N. Blood flow in the human Achilles tendon assessed by laser Doppler flowmetry. J Orthop Res 1994;12(2):246–52.

Anatomy: Plantar Plate

Daniel J. Hatch, DPM,FACFAS

KEYWORDS

- Plantar plate • Fibrocartilage • Accessory collateral ligament

KEY POINTS

- The plantar plate provides stability to the MTP.
- The plate resists tension forces.
- Composition of the plate also allows it to resist compression forces.

INTRODUCTION

Although the metatarsophalangeal (MTP) joints in the foot all have a plantar plate, the this discussion focuses on the lesser MTP joints, especially the second. It is at this joint that biomechanical factors frequently interplay resulting in sometimes acute, but mostly chronic overload-type injuries to the plantar plate. The anatomic influences of the plantar plate are discussed and illustrated to help provide a better understanding of the pathomechanics and subsequent repair options.

DISCUSSION

The plantar plate is a fibrocartilaginous structure extending from the periosteum of the inferior metatarsal neck to the inferior aspect of the base of the proximal phalanx. The plantar plate is composed mostly of type 1 (75%) and type 2 (21%) collagen.[1] The plantar plate has several important functions about the MTP. The main function of the plantar plate offers stability to the MTP[2–4]; this is due to the plantar plate and multiple attachments. In addition, the plantar plate offers a compression dampening at the MTP with weight-bearing forces due to its fibrocartilaginous composition.[1,2,5] The plantar plate also affords resistance to tensile forces as related to the windlass effect with the proximal attachment of the plantar fascia and subsequent dorsiflexion of the MTP.[2,6]

The second MTP joint is the most common location where a plantar plate injury may occur.[7] Lesser MTP tears have been reported in more than 40% of those with metatarsalgia and in 90% at the second MTP joint.[8] Coughlin[9] reported a 90% incidence of long second metatarsal with second toe crossover deformity. Nery and colleagues[10]

Director of Surgery, North Colorado Podiatric Medical Surgical Residency, 1931 65th Avenue, Suite A, Greeley, CO 80634, USA
E-mail address: djhdpm@gmail.com

Clin Podiatr Med Surg 39 (2022) 411–419
https://doi.org/10.1016/j.cpm.2022.02.004
0891-8422/22/© 2022 Elsevier Inc. All rights reserved.

podiatric.theclinics.com

found that the second MTP was involved in 63% of their cases followed by the third MTP (34%) and the fourth MTP at 3%. Most investigators agree that the plantar plate is the primary stabilizing structure and the first to fail,[7,11] and this is then followed by the collateral ligaments as the pathomechanics advances.

The origin of the plantar plate has been described by a couple of investigators. Johnston and colleagues[1] described it as being a fibrous, loose synovial-type attachment.[2] The thickness at this origin was approximately 0.4 mm compared with the main thickness of the plantar plate of 2 to 5 mm^2 (**Fig. 1**). This attachment site is augmented by the attachment of the distal slips of the plantar fascia[12] (**Fig. 2**A and B). In addition, the collateral ligaments and the deep transverse metatarsal ligaments (DTMLs) attach to this area.[2] This combination of origin attachments offers a secure proximal anchor (**Fig. 3**).

There are multiple attachments to the plantar plate mostly at its proximal two-thirds.[2] There are 2 collateral ligaments on the side of the MTP. Kelikian and Sarrafian[13] describe these as the metatarsophalangeal ligament and metatarsosesamoid (suspensory) ligament. More recent investigators describe these as the proper collateral and accessory collateral ligament (ACL)[2,14] (**Fig. 4**). The proper collateral goes from the epicondyle of the metatarsal to the inferior aspect of the proximal phalanx. The ACL goes from the epicondylar ridge of the metatarsal to the plantar plate (**Fig. 5**). The collaterals offer significant stability to this joint complex. Bhatia and colleagues[15] studied 25 cadaveric specimens and determined the load to displace the MTP in the vertical plane by 2.5 mm. Release of the plantar plate decreased the load needed to displace by 30%. The release of the collaterals reduced the load needed by 46% (**Fig. 6**). Suero and colleagues[11] studied 54 feet and applied a 30 N force across the joint to test stability. The investigators found the release of the plantar plate reduced stability by 19%. Release of the collaterals reduced stability by 37%. Release of both plantar plate and collaterals resulted in a 63% reduction in sagittal plane stability. Barg and colleagues[3] studied the effects of the collaterals on the MTP stability. The investigators studied 26 feet and determined the force needed to displace the joint by 3 mm. Their conclusion was that the ACL provided the greatest stability to the joint resisting vertical displacement.

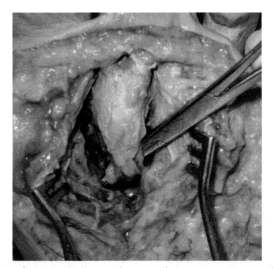

Fig. 1. Plantar view of proximal plantar plate attachment into metatarsal.

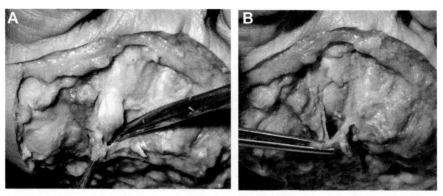

Fig. 2. (*A*) Plantar fascia inserting into plantar plate with flexor tendons intact. (*B*) Flexor tendons removed showing bipennant insertion into plate and deep transverse metatarsal ligament.

The DTML also provides significant stability to this joint complex. The combination of the plantar plate, DTML, and collaterals forms a transverse tie-bar system that provides transverse plane stability to the foot[5,16] (**Fig. 7**). Various investigators have discussed the importance of the DTML as related to sagittal stability of the MTP. Wang

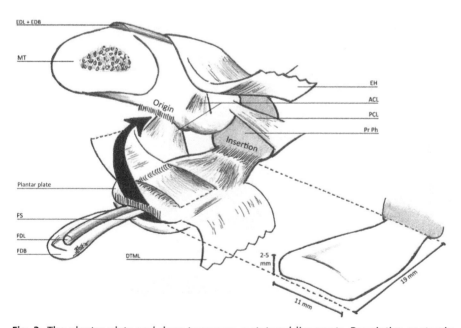

Fig. 3. The plantar plate and deep transverse metatarsal ligaments. Descriptive anatomic and histologic data visualized in a schematic 3D drawing of the PP. ACL, accessory collateral ligament; DTML, deep transverse metatarsal ligament; EDL + EDB, extensor digitorum longus/brevis; EH, extensor hood; FDL + FDB, flexor digitorum longus/brevis; FS, flexor sheath; MT, metatarsal; PCL, proper collateral ligament; Pr Ph, proximal phalanx. (*From* Maas NM, van der Grinten M, Bramer WM, Kleinrensink GJ. Metatarsophalangeal joint stability: a systematic review on the plantar plate of the lesser toes. J Foot Ankle Res. 2016 Aug 19;9:32. https://doi.org/10.1186/s13047-016-0165-2. PMID: 27547243; PMCID: PMC4992309.)

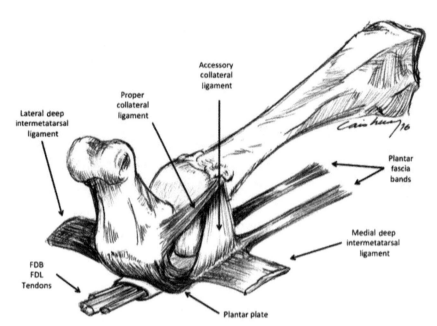

Fig. 4. Collateral ligaments with plantar plate and deep intermetatarsal ligament. (*From* Nery C, Baumfeld D, Umans H, Yamada AF. MR Imaging of the Plantar Plate: Normal Anatomy, Turf Toe, and Other Injuries. Magn Reson Imaging Clin N Am. 2017 Feb;25(1):127-144. https://doi.org/10.1016/j.mric.2016.08.007. PMID: 27888844.)

and colleagues[17] evaluated the second, third, and fourth MTP of 6 cadaveric specimens and determined the mean stiffness for dorsiflexion of the joint. With transection of one adjacent DTML the stiffness decreased 16.1%. Further transection of the other side DTML resulted in an additional decrease of 7.6%. Their summary indicated that the DTML provided a natural restraint to dorsiflexion and dorsal subluxation of the MTP.

The importance of the collaterals and DTML was nicely summarized in a systematic review published by Maas and colleagues[6] in 2016.

Additional attachments to the plantar plate may also include the interosseous tendons and the fibrous sheath of the flexor tendons (**Fig. 8**). The first lumbrical may

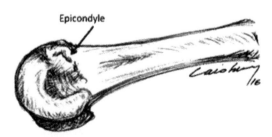

Fig. 5. Epicondylar ridge where collaterals attach. (*From* Nery C, Baumfeld D, Umans H, Yamada AF. MR Imaging of the Plantar Plate: Normal Anatomy, Turf Toe, and Other Injuries. Magn Reson Imaging Clin N Am. 2017 Feb;25(1):127-144. https://doi.org/10.1016/j.mric. 2016.08.007. PMID: 27888844.)

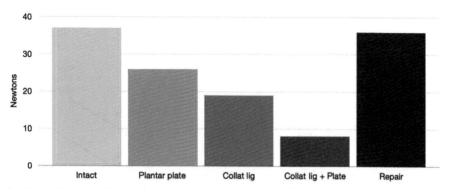

Fig. 6. Load required to displace joint by 2.5 mm. Note the flexor transfer repair after transection of plate and collaterals resulted in near-normal levels.

have some attachments to the distal plantar plate. One theory for the development of a crossover hammertoe is the unopposed medial attachment of the lumbrical.[18] Additionally some plantar interossei fibers may attach to the plate as well.[1] Deland and colleagues[19] proposed a proximal transfer of a section of the dorsal interossei into the neck of the metatarsal for surgical repair. The investigators stated that this works by the distal attachments into the inferior of the base of the proximal phalanx and plantar plate. Deland and colleagues[2] also reported on a unique ligamentous attachment from the distal lateral aspect of the plantar plate to the lateral aspect of the proximal phalanx. This attachment measured 3 to 4 mm in length and less than 0.5 mm thick.

Overall, the attachments to the plantar plate include the following structures: collateral ligaments, DTML, plantar fascia, fibrous sheath of flexors, some interossei tendons, and the lumbrical.

The midsubstance portion of the plantar plate is described as being rectangular to trapezoidal. Johnston and colleagues[1] performed anatomic evaluations of the plantar plate in 20 cadaveric specimens. Mean dimensions were 19 mm long, 11 mm wide, and 2 to 5 mm thickness.[1] These dimensions were verified by Deland and colleagues[2] with a mean length of 20 mm and thickness of 2 to 4 mm (**Figs. 9** and **10**). The borders of the plantar plate have been reported as thicker than the central aspect.[1] The inferior aspect of the plantar plate has a fibrous groove for flexor tendons.

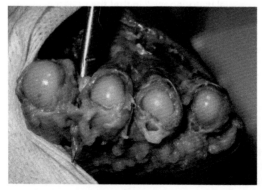

Fig. 7. Tie-bar system with plantar plate, collaterals. and DTML. Note tunnel where flexor tendon lies below the fourth metatarsal plantar plate (first metatarsal is removed).

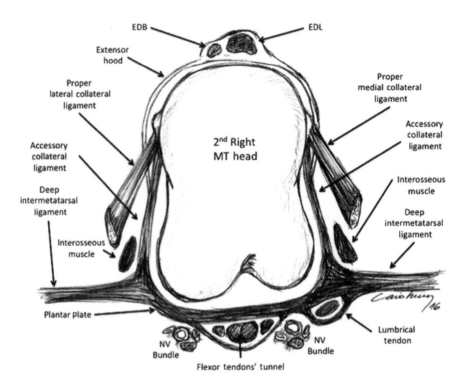

Fig. 8. Coronal section of the plantar plate at the metatarsal head showing the relationships of the intrinsic muscles and DTML. MT, metatarsal. (*From* Nery C, Baumfeld D, Umans H, Yamada AF. MR Imaging of the Plantar Plate: Normal Anatomy, Turf Toe, and Other Injuries. Magn Reson Imaging Clin N Am. 2017 Feb;25(1):127-144. https://doi.org/10.1016/j.mric.2016.08.007. PMID: 27888844.)

The distal enthesis of the plantar plate is securely attached to the inferior aspect of the base of the proximal phalanx. The stronger attachments seem to be on the perimeter.[2]

Histologic examination of the plate has also been evaluated by various investigators.[1,2,5] Gregg and colleagues[5] dedicated their research to the histologic evaluation of the plantar plate in longitudinal and transverse sections. The investigators reference Pauwel's theory of "casual histogenesis" in that the collagen fibrils will line up with the greatest tension. As such, in the dorsal two-thirds of the plate the collagen fibrils line up longitudinally with the tensile pull of the plantar fascia and dorsiflexion of the toe. More proximally, along the lower one-third, the fibrils line up transversely correlating the forces induced by the DTMLs. The investigators also found the proximal plate has higher amounts of chondrocytes (fibrocartilage), whereas the distal portion was more fibroblasts. It was summarized that the morphology of the plate correlates with forces applied at specific levels. The insertional fibers are under more tension and hence mostly ligamentous-type fibrous tissue. The midsubstance fibers are influenced more by compressive loads and are more fibrocartilaginous in structure. Gregg and colleagues[5] also found that vascular tissue seemed to enter on the peripheral aspect of the plate mainly plantarly. Further studies to elucidate the vascular influences on the plantar plate will provide more information for surgical repair such as Finney and colleagues.[20] The investigators uses nano-computed tomographic technology to evaluate the vascular influences along the course of the plantar plate.

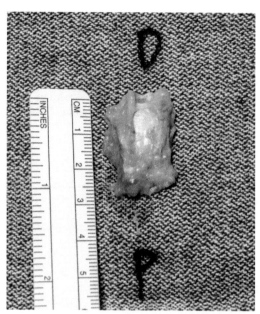

Fig. 9. Plantar view of plantar plate. Distal is at top of the photograph. Note central groove for flexor sheath.

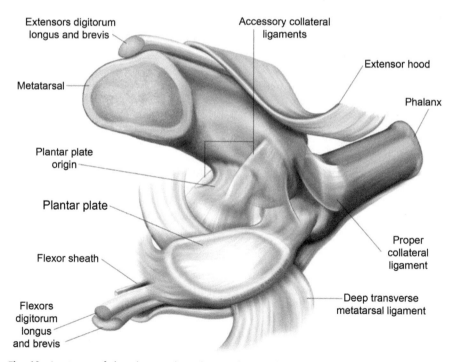

Fig. 10. Anatomy of the plantar plate. (*From* Chris Mallac, Plantar plate tear: a common overload injury in athletes, Ankle and foot injuries, Diagnose & Treat, https://www.sportsinjurybulletin.com/plantar-plate-tear-a-common-overload-injury-in-athletes/, with permission.)

They found an area of hypovascularity in the midsubstance of the plate, whereas more vascularity was noted proximally and distally at the attachment.

SUMMARY

The fibrocartilaginous composition of the plantar plate offers resistance to tension and compression forces at the MTP joints. It also provides the stability of the joint in conjunction with the plantar fascia, collateral ligaments, DTMLs, intrinsics muscles, and the flexor tendon sheath.

CLINICS CARE POINTS

- The synergistic effects of the plantar plate and collateral ligaments may necessitate concomitant repair when deficiency is noted.

DISCLOSURE

The author has nothing to disclose.

REFERENCES

1. Johnston RB 3rd, Smith J, Daniels T. The plantar plate of the lesser toes: an anatomical study in human cadavers. Foot Ankle Int 1994;15(5):276–82.
2. Deland JT, Lee KT, Sobel M, et al. Anatomy of the plantar plate and its attachments in the lesser metatarsal phalangeal joint. Foot Ankle Int 1995;16(8):480–6.
3. Barg A, Courville XF, Nickisch F, et al. Role of collateral ligaments in metatarsophalangeal stability: a cadaver study. Foot Ankle Int 2012;33(10):877–82.
4. Chalayon O, Chertman C, Guss AD, et al. Role of plantar plate and surgical reconstruction techniques on static stability of lesser metatarsophalangeal joints: a biomechanical study. Foot Ankle Int 2013;34(10):1436–42.
5. Gregg J, Marks P, Silberstein M, et al. Histologic anatomy of the lesser metatarsophalangeal joint plantar plate. Surg Radiol Anat 2007;29(2):141–7.
6. Maas NMG, van der Grinten M, Bramer WM, et al. Metatarsophalangeal joint stability: a systematic review on the plantar plate of the lesser toes. J Foot Ankle Res 2016;9:32.
7. Doty JF, Coughlin MJ. Metatarsophalangeal joint instability of the lesser toes and plantar plate deficiency. J Am Acad Orthop Surg 2014;22(4):235–45.
8. Umans H, Srinivasan R, Elsinger E, et al. MRI of lesser metatarsophalangeal joint plantar plate tears and associated adjacent interspace lesions. Skeletal Radiol 2014;43(10):1361–8.
9. Coughlin MJ. Crossover second toe deformity. Foot Ankle 1987;8(1):29–39.
10. Nery C, Coughlin MJ, Baumfeld D, et al. Prospective evaluation of protocol for surgical treatment of lesser MTP joint plantar plate tears. Foot Ankle Int 2014; 35(9):876–85.
11. Suero EM, Meyers KN, Bohne WHO. Stability of the metatarsophalangeal joint of the lesser toes: a cadaveric study. J Orthop Res 2012;30(12):1995–8.
12. Bojsen-Moller F, Flagstad KE. Plantar aponeurosis and internal architecture of the ball of the foot. J Anat 1976;121(Pt 3):599–611.
13. Kelikian AS, Sarrafian SK. Sarrafian's anatomy of the foot and ankle: descriptive, topographic, functional. Philadelphia (PA): Lippincott Williams & Wilkins; 2011.

14. Nery C, Baumfeld D, Umans H, et al. MR Imaging of the plantar plate: normal anatomy, turf toe, and other injuries. Magn Reson Imaging Clin N Am 2017; 25(1):127–44.

15. Bhatia D, Myerson MS, Curtis MJ, et al. Anatomical restraints to dislocation of the second metatarsophalangeal joint and assessment of a repair technique. J Bone Joint Surg Am 1994;76(9):1371–5.

16. Stainsby GD. Pathological anatomy and dynamic effect of the displaced plantar plate and the importance of the integrity of the plantar plate-deep transverse metatarsal ligament tie-bar. Ann R Coll Surg Engl 1997;79(1):58–68.

17. Wang B, Guss A, Chalayon O, et al. Deep transverse metatarsal ligament and static stability of lesser metatarsophalangeal joints: a cadaveric study. Foot Ankle Int 2015;36(5):573–8.

18. Doty JF, Coughlin MJ, Weil L Jr, et al. Etiology and management of lesser toe metatarsophalangeal joint instability. Foot Ankle Clin 2014;19(3):385–405.

19. Deland JT, Sobel M, Arnoczky SP, et al. Collateral Ligament reconstruction of the unstable metatarsophalangeal joint: an in vitro study. Foot Ankle 1992;13(7): 391–5.

20. Finney FT, McPheters A, Singer NV, et al. Microvasculature of the plantar plate using nano-computed tomography. Foot Ankle Int 2019;40(4):457–64.

Normal and Diseased Imaging: Ultrasound/MRI

Adam E. Fleischer, DPM, MPH, FACFAS[a,c,*],
Rachel H. Albright, DPM, MPH, AACFAS[b]

KEYWORDS

- Plantar plate • Volar plate • Flexor plate • Calcaneonavicular ligament
- Spring ligament

KEY POINTS

- Both MRI and diagnostic ultrasound are useful in the diagnosis of plantar plate pathology.
- Due to its high sensitivity and wide availability, point-of-care ultrasound can be used to rapidly rule out plantar plate pathology in clinical settings.
- Patients requiring further interrogation of the plantar plate may benefit from further testing with MRI to better quantify and localize pathology, and to assess the joint collateral ligaments.
- When advanced injuries of the plantar plate or spring ligament are suspected, fat-suppressed MR images help to determine just how much native collagen is still present in the area.
- In cases where little healthy collagen remains, a nonatomic repair or the addition of suture tape augmentation may be preferable to direct repair alone.

INTRODUCTION

Plantar plate injury and subluxation of the lesser metatarsophalangeal (MTP) joint is a relatively common phenomenon,[1–3] and growing attention has been given to this problem in recent years; this is evidenced by the 5-fold increase in the number of publications with "plantar plate" in their title in just the past 5 years alone. Although it is well known that injuries to the fibrocartilaginous plantar plate allow for the advancement of hammertoe deformities,[3,4] these injuries have also become increasingly recognized for their role as pain generators within the forefoot.[5,6] As a result, surgical repair of the tissue has become an increasingly more common practice among foot and ankle surgeons around the world.[2] Preoperative ultrasound and MRI can help with

[a] Weil Foot & Ankle Institute, 3000 N, Halsted Suite 700, Chicago, IL 60657, USA; [b] Stamford Health Medical Group, 800 Boston Post Road, Suite 302, Darien, CT 06820, USA; [c] Dr. William M. Scholl College of Podiatric Medicine, Rosalind Franklin University of Medicine and Science, North Chicago, IL 60064, USA
* Corresponding author. Weil Foot & ankle Institute, 3000 N. Halsted Suite 700, Chicago, IL 60657.
E-mail address: aef@weil4feet.com

Clin Podiatr Med Surg 39 (2022) 421–435
https://doi.org/10.1016/j.cpm.2022.03.004

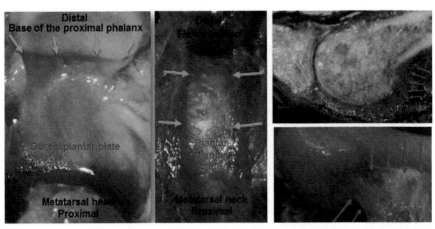

Fig. 1. Typical dorsal and plantar appearance of the plantar plate along with its distal (*green arrows*) and proximal attachments (*pink arrows*). The dorsal surface of the plantar plate has an articularlike appearance and is composed primarily of type 1 collagen, which resembles fibrocartilage.[32–34] The plantar third of the plantar plate has fibers that are organized in a transverse fashion to facilitate the attachments of the plantar plate to the deep transverse metatarsal ligament and is adjacent to the long flexor tendon and its tendon sheath.[32–35]

identifying the presence and magnitude of plantar plate injuries and play a role in directing procedure selection (eg, direct repair of the plate, direct repair with suture tape augmentation, or indirect/nonanatomic repair with flexor digitorum longus tendon transfer).

Similarly, there is also growing interest within the foot and ankle surgical community in the foot's other fibrocartilaginous support—the calcaneonavicular (spring) ligament. Acting as a sling for the talar head, the spring ligament is the primary support of the medial arch and is therefore commonly found to be incompetent in cases of acquired flatfoot deformity where the posterior tibialis tendon is dysfunctional.[7] Chronic laxity of the spring ligament leads to plantarflexion of the talar head further propagating a planovalgus foot structure.[8] Given its important structural and biomechanical function, repair or reconstruction (with and without suture tape augmentation) of the spring ligament has become an evolving consideration as an adjunct procedure during surgical

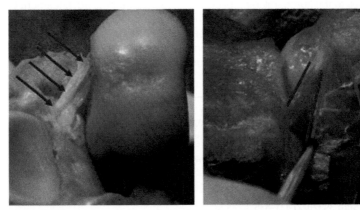

Fig. 2. The suspensory (*pink lines*) and collateral (*blue arrows/lines*) ligaments of the lesser MTP joint.

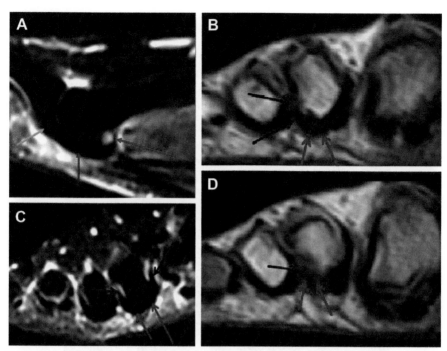

Fig. 3. (*A*) The plantar plate (*pink arrow*) seems hypointense on MRI and has a stout distal attachment (*green arrow*) with a proximal attachment that tapers and blends with the periosteum of the metatarsal (*red arrow*). (*B*) Collateral ligaments (*blue arrows*) should seem black and taut on the coronal images. (*C, D*) Coronal MR images depicting a lateral collateral ligament tear (*blue arrows*) with disruption of the lateral plantar plate (*pink arrows*).

treatment of flatfoot deformity. Preoperatively, advanced imaging can be used to determine the extent of spring ligament injury and, just as in plantar plate pathology, subsequently aid in procedure (and material) selection.

This article focuses on ultrasound and MRI—the 2 modalities commonly used to image the fibrocartilaginous lesser MTP joint plantar plate and spring ligament. Technical considerations and a description of normal and abnormal appearances are provided. The pros and cons of each imaging modality are also discussed in the context of plantar plate and spring ligament pathology.

PLANTAR PLATE

Advanced imaging is indispensable for surgeons hoping to both confirm and better localize plantar plate injuries.[9] It can also provide insight into the magnitude of injury (and therefore the presence/absence of remaining native collagen) and provide important information regarding the integrity of the joint's supporting structures, such as the collateral ligaments. The gross appearance of the lesser MTP joint plantar plate can be seen in (**Fig. 1**). Similar to the plantar plate, the collateral ligaments also play a *critical role* in stabilizing the lesser MTP joint in the sagittal plane.[10] In fact, cadaveric studies have found that sectioning of (1) only the plantar plate, (2) only the collateral ligaments, and (3) both the plantar plate and collateral ligaments decreases the amount of force needed to dislocate the second MTP joint by 30%, 46%, and 80%, respectively.[10] The medial and lateral collateral MTP ligaments course anterior and inferiorly to attach to

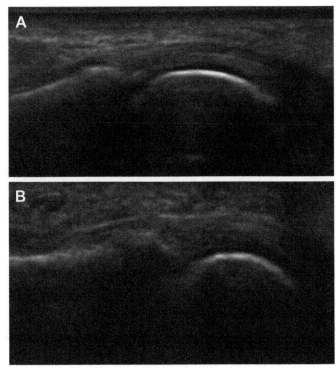

Fig. 4. (*A*) The plantar plate normally seems taut and echogenic on diagnostic ultrasound longitudinal scans. (*B*) When injured, it can seem thickened and hypoechoic with distortion of the overlying long flexor tendon as seen here.

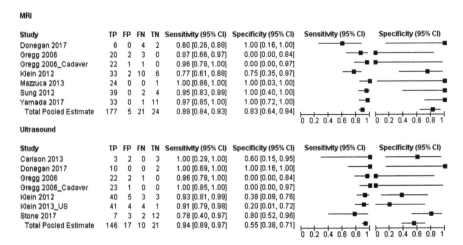

MRI

Study	TP	FP	FN	TN	Sensitivity (95% CI)	Specificity (95% CI)
Donegan 2017	6	0	4	2	0.60 [0.26, 0.88]	1.00 [0.16, 1.00]
Gregg 2006	20	2	3	0	0.87 [0.66, 0.97]	0.00 [0.00, 0.84]
Gregg 2006_Cadaver	22	1	1	0	0.96 [0.78, 1.00]	0.00 [0.00, 0.97]
Klein 2012	33	2	10	6	0.77 [0.61, 0.88]	0.75 [0.35, 0.97]
Mazzuca 2013	24	0	0	1	1.00 [0.86, 1.00]	1.00 [0.03, 1.00]
Sung 2012	39	0	2	4	0.95 [0.83, 0.99]	1.00 [0.40, 1.00]
Yamada 2017	33	0	1	11	0.97 [0.85, 1.00]	1.00 [0.72, 1.00]
Total Pooled Estimate	177	5	21	24	0.89 [0.84, 0.93]	0.83 [0.64, 0.94]

Ultrasound

Study	TP	FP	FN	TN	Sensitivity (95% CI)	Specificity (95% CI)
Carlson 2013	3	2	0	3	1.00 [0.29, 1.00]	0.60 [0.15, 0.95]
Donegan 2017	10	0	0	2	1.00 [0.69, 1.00]	1.00 [0.16, 1.00]
Gregg 2006	22	2	1	0	0.96 [0.78, 1.00]	0.00 [0.00, 0.84]
Gregg 2006_Cadaver	23	1	0	0	1.00 [0.85, 1.00]	0.00 [0.00, 0.97]
Klein 2012	40	5	3	3	0.93 [0.81, 0.99]	0.38 [0.09, 0.76]
Klein 2013_US	41	4	4	1	0.91 [0.79, 0.98]	0.20 [0.01, 0.72]
Stone 2017	7	3	2	12	0.78 [0.40, 0.97]	0.80 [0.52, 0.96]
Total Pooled Estimate	146	17	10	21	0.94 [0.89, 0.97]	0.55 [0.38, 0.71]

Fig. 5. MRI versus ultrasound in the diagnosis of plantar plate tears. Forest plots demonstrating the summary estimates for sensitivity and specificity for each modality. FN, false negative; FP, false positive; TN, true negative; TP, true positive.

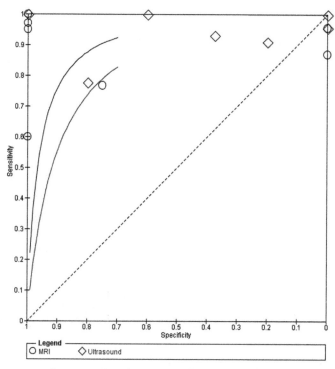

Fig. 6. Summary receiver operating characteristic (ROC) curves for diagnosing plantar plate tears. MRI performs slightly better than ultrasound (US) in overall accuracy.

the plantar-medial and plantar-lateral portions of the base of the proximal phalanx, respectively, in close proximity to the plantar plate[11] (**Fig. 2**). Therefore, when interrogating plantar plate injuries with advanced imaging, it is important to describe not only the integrity of the fibrocartilaginous plantar plate but also the integrity of the joint's supporting collateral ligaments, when able.

MRI

High-resolution positioning coils should be used to enhance anatomic detail in the lesser MTP joints when available. Although all MRI planes will be helpful, the coronal slices typically provide the best and most direct visualization of the plantar plate. The collateral ligaments, similarly, are best seen on coronal (and occasionally axial) images. Sagittal images will be less useful when looking for plantar plate injuries and tears, unless the injury is extensive.[12]

Similar to all dense collagen, the normal plantar plate appears hypointense (black) and uniform (homogenous) on MRI. It has a stout distal attachment with a tapering proximal attachment that blends with the periosteum of the metatarsal. The collateral ligaments, when uninjured, appear black and taut on the coronal images on all sequences. Disruptions (eg, ruptures and tears) within the plantar plate, on the other hand, are evidenced by focal areas of intermediate signal intensity and will be best visualized on coronal images taken through the joint. These are frequently accompanied by a wavy or disrupted medial or lateral collateral ligament (**Fig. 3**). In advanced injuries, it is important to look closely at the fat-suppressed images (eg, typically the T2

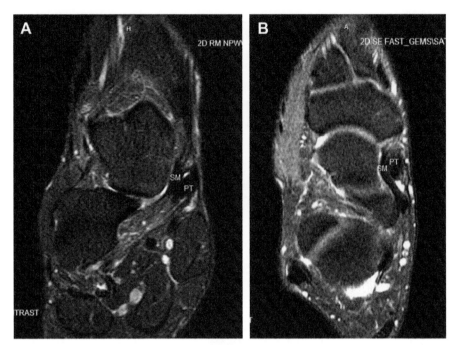

Fig. 7. Coronal (*A*) and axial (*B*) T2-weighted images demonstrating the close relationship of the superomedial (SM) portion of the spring ligament with the posterior tibialis tendon (PT). The normal appearance of the SM spring ligament is black, homogenous, of uniform thickness, and taut.

sequences) to determine just how much native collagen is still present in the area. Remaining viable collagen will appear black on T2-weighted images. In cases where little black collagen remains, a nonanatomic repair (eg, flexor to extensor tendon transfer) or augmented repair (eg, with suture tape) may be preferable to a direct/primary repair. In patients with more subtle pathology and attenuation only of the plate, sometimes the only MRI evidence will be a slightly nonhomogenous appearing plantar plate and/or small effusion or focal subcutaneous edema located at the plantar lateral aspect of the joint.[13]

Ultrasound Imaging

Ultrasound examination of the plantar plate has gained significant attention in recent years. The distinct advantages are that ultrasound can be performed at the point of care, and it allows the examiner, many times the surgeon him or herself, to perform drawer testing (dynamic testing) with direct visualization of the plantar plate during provocation. Visualization of the planter plate should be performed in both longitudinal and transverse (short) axes with a plantar approach. The base of the proximal phalanx is the most common location for plantar plate injury and should therefore be scanned carefully. The plantar plate is normally taut and echogenic (bright and fibrillar) on diagnostic ultrasound scans. When injured, it usually seems thickened and hypoechoic (black) with distortion of the overlying long flexor tendon (**Fig. 4**). Dorsiflexion of the MTP joint helps to identify attenuation and/or tears within the planter plate and is best performed while scanning in long axis. An unstable plantar plate can be readily identified by performing a dynamic Lachman test under direct ultrasound visualization.

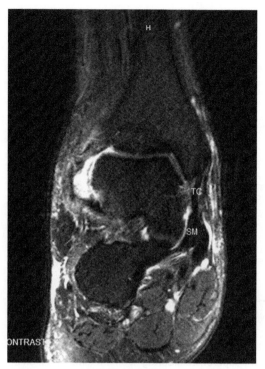

Fig. 8. A normal-appearing superomedial spring ligament (SM) blending superiorly with the tibiocalcaneal ligament (TC), part of the superficial deltoid. Together these form the primary static stabilization of the foot's medial longitudinal arch.

This test consists of the clinician stabilizing the metatarsal and translating the proximal phalanx dorsally to assess laxity of the plantar plate. Real-time sonographic imaging can provide visual confirmation of joint laxity even in subtle cases of joint instability when the clinical maneuver is negative or equivocal. With full-thickness tears, many times a small joint effusion, or herniation of fluid, will be seen extravasating out from the plantar joint while the examiner holds the toe in extension, and this effusion then goes away on relaxation/reduction of the joint.

MRI Versus Ultrasound Debate for Plantar Plate Injuries

Our group recently performed a systematic review and meta-analysis of MEDLINE and CINAHL databases to examine the diagnostic performance of MRI and ultrasound for plantar plate injuries.[14] We followed standard methodology for performing a meta-analysis using the Preferred Reporting Items for Systematic Reviews and Meta-Analyses (PRISMA) guidelines. Inclusion criteria included any original study that was published in a peer-reviewed journal that tested the diagnostic accuracy for detecting a plantar plate tear using MRI or ultrasound. Studies were included if they reported on the sensitivity and specificity of one or more of the aforementioned tests. Visual inspection of the plantar plate (during open surgery or arthroscopically) was used as the reference/gold standard. Sensitivity and specificity were obtained and, when possible, pooled from included studies. Summary receiver operating characteristic curves were formed for diagnostic tests to compare accuracy. Study quality was assessed using the QUADAS scoring system.

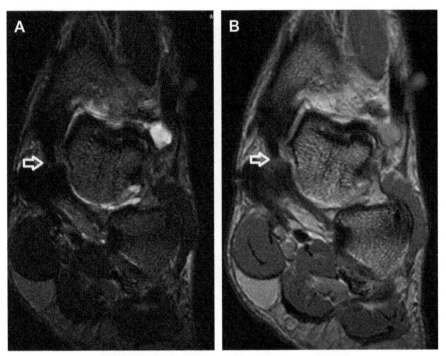

Fig. 9. A rupture of the superomedial spring ligament (SM) is seen on both T2-weighted coronal images (*A*) and proton dense images (*B*) with complete disruption occurring at the confluence of the SM and tibiocalcaneal ligaments (*arrow*).

One thousand seven hundred fifteen unique articles were initially identified, and 10 studies[9,15–23] met our inclusion criteria, representing 227 plantar plates for MRI and 194 plantar plates for ultrasound. The overall study quality was good, with generally low (n = 6) or medium (n = 3) risk for bias across the included studies. MRI displayed a pooled sensitivity of 89% (95% confidence interval [CI] 0.84, 0.93) and pooled specificity of 83% (95% CI 0.64, 0.94). Ultrasound displayed a pooled sensitivity and pooled specificity of 94% (95% CI 0.89, 0.97) and 55% (95% CI 0.38, 0.71), respectively (**Fig. 5**). Overall, the diagnostic accuracy of MRI was slightly better than that of ultrasound (**Fig. 6**).

Our takeaway was that both MRI and dynamic ultrasound can be useful in the diagnosis of plantar plate pathology. The clear advantage to ultrasound is that it can be performed at the point of care, and it allows the examiner (many times the surgeon him or herself) to perform drawer testing with direct visualization of the plantar plate itself during provocation.[24] In contrast, MRI seems to be a slightly more accurate method overall for diagnosing plantar plate pathology while providing insight into the integrity of the joint's additional supporting structures (eg, collateral ligaments), which ultrasound is not capable of.

In our practice, due to its high sensitivity, we use dynamic, in-office ultrasound during the patient encounter to rule out injuries to the plantar plate. In the case of an equivocal or positive ultrasound examination, we then refer the patient for a dedicated forefoot MRI to evaluate the plantar plate more specifically (including its native collagen) and to further assess the associated collateral ligaments.

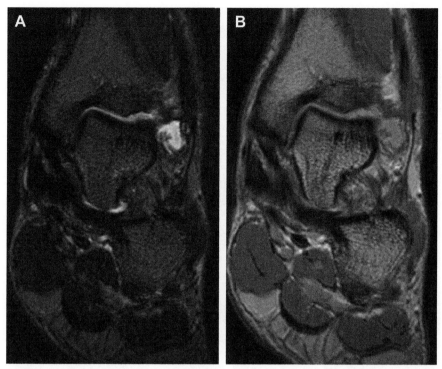

Fig. 10. A chronic tear of the superomedial spring ligament is seen here on both T2-weighted coronal images (A) and proton dense images (B) with distortion (thickening and increased heterogeneity) of the normally black and homogenous collagen.

SPRING LIGAMENT

The spring ligament, also referred to as the calcaneonavicular ligament, is commonly injured in adult-acquired flatfoot deformity. The broad ligamentous complex is often divided into upper, medial, and lower regions and frequently described as having a superomedial (SM) ligament, an inferior ligament, and a medioplantar oblique (MPO) ligament. The SM ligament is a broad rectangular segment of the spring ligament that originates from the anterior and medial aspects of the sustentaculum tali and the anterior margin of the articular surface of the calcaneus.[8] Oriented anteriorly, the SM ligament inserts at the margin of the posterior articular surface of the navicular. It is the medial portion of the SM ligament that follows closely with the posterior tibialis tendon. The lateral portion of the SM ligament articulates with the head of the talus. The inferior ligament supports the inferior portion of the talus. It originates from the coronoid fossa between the middle and anterior facets of the calcaneus and courses medially, inserting on the plantar aspect of the navicular where it meets the SM ligament.[8] The MPO ligament shares the same origin as the inferior ligament; however, the MPO ligament inserts at the inferior and medial portions of the navicular, whereas the inferior ligament inserts at the lateral and inferior portions.[25] Although earlier texts describe the spring ligament in 2 distinct regions (SM and inferior ligaments only), several radiographical studies have successfully identified the 3 distinct portions of the spring ligament.[25–27]

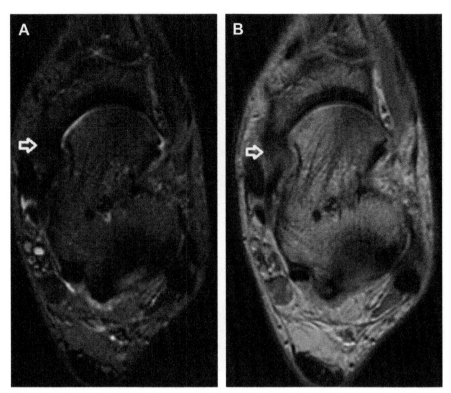

Fig. 11. On axial images, a chronic tear of the superomedial spring ligament is frequently seen as thickening and heterogeneity of the ligament (*arrow*) adjacent to the talar head and navicular insertion. (*A*) T2-weighted axial images; (*B*) proton dense axial images.

MRI

MRI is a valuable modality for diagnosing spring ligament injuries because it provides visualization of the structures in multiple planes. It also allows for evaluation of related conditions (eg, tarsal coalition) and commonly associated soft tissue injuries (eg, tibio-calcaneal [superficial deltoid] ligament injuries and posterior tibialis tendon injuries). Given the SM ligament represents the broadest portion of the spring ligament, it is the easiest portion to identify pathology via imaging.

The SM spring ligament is best visualized in the coronal and axial planes (**Fig. 7**). When uninjured, the normal SM ligament can be seen on coronal images blending superiorly with the tibiocalcaneal ligament (also called the tibiospring ligament), which forms part of the superficial deltoid ligament complex (**Fig. 8**). Ruptures of the SM spring ligament are evidenced by a disruption in this relationship (**Fig. 9**), and chronic tears frequently manifest as distortions (thickening and increased heterogeneity) of the ligament (**Figs. 10** and **11**). The most common finding on MRI of an injured spring ligament is high/intermediate signal intensity on proton dense images or T2-weighted images and discontinuity of the SM ligament in the presence of acquired flatfoot deformity. One radiographic study examining 43 injured spring ligaments via MRI versus 29 healthy controls recorded 77% of their injured population displayed high signal intensity of the SM on MRI and 47% displayed discontinuity of the SM on MRI. Waviness of the SM ligament was also reported on MRI; however, the investigators noted this

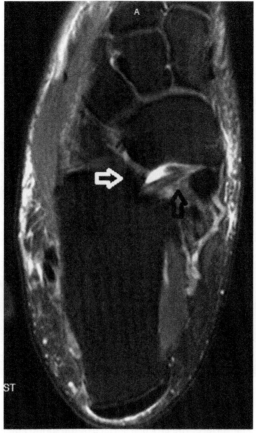

Fig. 12. The medioplantar oblique (*black arrow*) and inferior (*white arrow*) ligaments of the spring complex can be well visualized on fat-saturated proton dense axial images.

finding was less predictable with only 35% of the cohort displaying this characteristic when spring ligament injury was present.[28]

The MPO ligament is the thinnest portion of the spring ligament complex and may seem striated on T1 images; however, injuries to the MPO and inferior ligaments are rarely reported in the literature. The MPO and inferior ligaments are best visualized in the axial plane (**Fig. 12**).

Ultrasound Imaging

The spring ligament can be visualized with musculoskeletal ultrasound with sagittal oblique images. Similar ultrasound technique is generally agreed on within the literature.[29–31] The examiner should first palpate the anatomic landmarks of the sustentaculum tali and the navicular. The ultrasound probe can then be placed inferior to the medial malleolus with positioning of the probe over the sustentaculum tali and tilted superiorly over the talar head toward the navicular, parallel to the plantar aspect of the foot. Some reports have noted that the attachment of the spring ligament is not always well visualized. In those instances, the navicular tuberosity can be palpated and identified.[30,31] The probe can then be tilted slightly dorsal to visualize the dorsal

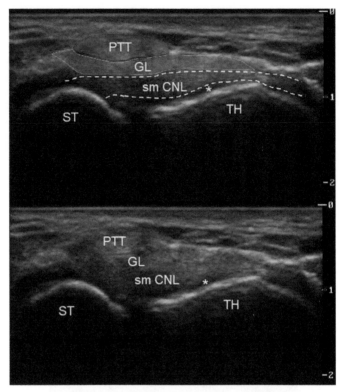

Fig. 13. Long-axis sonographic appearance of a normal spring ligament. The superomedial calcaneonavicular ligament (sm CNL) (*dotted line*) originates from the sustentaculum tali (ST) and passes over the talar head (TH). The inner portion of the superomedial CNL directly articulates with the talar surface. The articular surface of the spring ligament is covered with fibrocartilage (*asterisk*), creating an articular surface with the head of the talus. Between the superomedial CNL and the posterior tibialis tendon (PTT), there is a loose connective tissue layer that provides a gliding layer (GL).

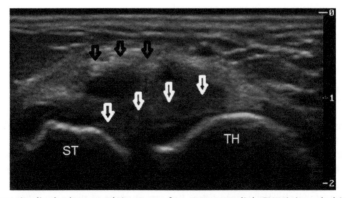

Fig. 14. Longitudinal ultrasound images of a superomedial CNL injury (*white arrows*) showing loss of the normal fibrillar echogenic pattern and mild thickening. Posterior tibialis tendon (*black arrows*) shows some mild hypoechoic tenosynovitis but is otherwise normal.

aspect of the navicular tuberosity, which may help aid in identifying the spring ligament coverage over the talar head. The normal SM portion of the spring ligament will seem hyperechoic with a fibrillar appearing pattern (**Fig. 13**). A diseased ligament will seem thickened, with loss of internal echoes and is occasionally accompanied by a talonavicular joint effusion on ranging of the subtalar and talonavicular joints (**Fig. 14**).

SUMMARY

Point-of-care ultrasound can effectively rule out a serious injury to the plantar plate and spring ligaments when the result is "normal." In cases of suspected pathology on ultrasound, further workup with MRI is typically a prudent next step due to its higher specificity and overall accuracy. When advanced injuries are suspected, it is important to examine the fat-suppressed MRI (eg, T2-weighted sequences) to determine just how much native (black-appearing) collagen is still present in the area. In cases where little healthy collagen remains, a nonatomic repair (eg, flexor to extensor tendon transfer) or the addition of suture tape augmentation may be preferable to direct repair alone.

CLINICS CARE POINTS

- Point-of-care ultrasound, when negative, rules out a serious injury to the plantar plate and spring ligaments.

- MRI, however, will be more accurate and specific in recognizing and quantifying plantar plate pathology than ultrasound.

- T2-weighted MR images can be used preoperatively to reliably identify scenarios where nonanatomic repair, or the addition of suture tape augmentation, may be preferable to direct repair alone.

REFERENCES

1. Coughlin MJ. Crossover second toe deformity. Foot Ankle 1987;8:29.
2. Doty JF, Coughlin MJ. Metatarsophalangeal joint instability of the lesser toes and plantar plate deficiency. J Am Acad Orthop Surg 2014;22:235.
3. Doty JF, Coughlin MJ, Weil L Jr, et al. Etiology and management of lesser toe metatarsophalangeal joint instability. Foot Ankle Clin 2014;19:385.
4. Coughlin MJ, Schutt SA, Hirose CB, et al. Metatarsophalangeal joint pathology in crossover second toe deformity: a cadaveric study. Foot Ankle Int 2012;33:133.
5. Bouché RT, Heit EJ. Combined plantar plate and hammertoe repair with flexor digitorum longus tendon transfer for chronic, severe sagittal plane instability of the lesser metatarsophalangeal joints: preliminary observations. J Foot Ankle Surg 2008;47:125.
6. Weil L Jr, Sung W, Weil LS, et al. Anatomic plantar plate repair using the Weil metatarsal osteotomy approach. Foot Ankle Spec 2011;4:145.
7. Domzalski M, Kwapisz A, Zabierek S. Morphology of spring ligament fibrocartilage complex lesions. J Am Podiatr Med Assoc 2019;109:407.
8. Bastias GF, Dalmau-Pastor M, Astudillo C, et al. Spring ligament instability. Foot Ankle Clin 2018;23:659.
9. Sung W, Weil L Jr, Weil LS Sr, et al. Diagnosis of plantar plate injury by magnetic resonance imaging with reference to intraoperative findings. J Foot Ankle Surg 2012;51:570.

10. Bhatia D, Myerson MS, Curtis MJ, et al. Anatomical restraints to dislocation of the second metatarsophalangeal joint and assessment of a repair technique. J Bone Joint Surg Am 1994;76:1371.

11. Sarrafian SK, Topouzian LK. Anatomy and physiology of the extensor apparatus of the toes. J Bone Joint Surg Am 1969;51:669.

12. Ormond Filho AGPD, Narahashi E, Nico MA. Unraveling the plantar plate in MRI: normal and pathologic findings. J Foot Ankle 2016;10:39.

13. Coughlin MJ, Baumfeld DS, Nery C. Second MTP joint instability: grading of the deformity and description of surgical repair of capsular insufficiency. Phys Sportsmed 2011;39:132.

14. Albright RH, Chingre M, Brooks B, et al. Diagnostic accuracy of magnetic resonance imaging (MRI) versus dynamic ultrasound for plantar plate injuries: a systematic review and meta-analysis. Eur J Radiol. In Press 2022.

15. Donegan RJ, Stauffer A, Heaslet M, et al. Comparing magnetic resonance imaging and high-resolution dynamic ultrasonography for diagnosis of plantar plate pathology: a case series. J Foot Ankle Surg 2017;56:371.

16. Gregg J, Silberstein M, Schneider T, et al. Sonographic and MRI evaluation of the plantar plate: a prospective study. Eur Radiol 2006;16:2661.

17. Gregg JM, Silberstein M, Schneider T, et al. Sonography of plantar plates in cadavers: correlation with MRI and histology. AJR Am J Roentgenol 2006;186:948.

18. Stone M, Eyler W, Rhodenizer J, et al. Accuracy of sonography in plantar plate tears in cadavers. J Ultrasound Med 2017;36:1355.

19. Klein EE, Weil L Jr, Weil LS, et al. Magnetic resonance imaging versus musculoskeletal ultrasound for identification and localization of plantar plate tears. Foot Ankle Spec 2012;5:359.

20. Klein EE, Weil L Jr, Weil LS, et al. Musculoskeletal ultrasound for preoperative imaging of the plantar plate: a prospective analysis. Foot Ankle Spec 2013;6:196.

21. Carlson RM, Dux K, Stuck RM. Ultrasound imaging for diagnosis of plantar plate ruptures of the lesser metatarsophalangeal joints: a retrospective case series. J Foot Ankle Surg 2013;52:786.

22. Mazzuca JW, Yonke B, Downes JM, et al. Flouroscopic arthrography versus MR arthrography of the lesser metatarsophalangeal joints for the detection of tears of the plantar plate and joint capsule: a prospective comparative study. Foot Ankle Int 2013;34:200.

23. Yamada AF, Crema MD, Nery C, et al. Second and third metatarsophalangeal plantar plate tears: diagnostic performance of direct and indirect mri features using surgical findings as the reference standard. AJR Am J Roentgenol 2017;209:W100.

24. Feuerstein CA, Weil L Jr, Weil LS Sr, et al. Static versus dynamic musculoskeletal ultrasound for detection of plantar plate pathology. Foot Ankle Spec 2014;7:259.

25. Mengiardi B, Pinto C, Zanetti M. Spring ligament complex and posterior tibial tendon: mr anatomy and findings in acquired adult flatfoot deformity. Semin Musculoskelet Radiol 2016;20:104.

26. Mansour R, Jibri Z, Kamath S, et al. Persistent ankle pain following a sprain: a review of imaging. Emerg Radiol 2011;18:211.

27. Szaro P, Ghali Gataa K, Ciszek B. Anatomical variants of the medioplantar oblique ligament and inferoplantar longitudinal ligament: an MRI study. Surg Radiol Anat 2022;44:279.

28. Kimura Y, Yamashiro T, Saito Y, et al. MRI findings of spring ligament injury: association with surgical findings and flatfoot deformity. Acta Radiol Open 2020;9. 2058460120980145.

29. Mansour R, Teh J, Sharp RJ, et al. Ultrasound assessment of the spring ligament complex. Eur Radiol 2008;18:2670.
30. Tanaka K, Kudo S. Functional assessment of the spring ligament using ultrasonography in the Japanese population. Foot (Edinb) 2020;44:101665.
31. Harish S, Jan E, Finlay K, et al. Sonography of the superomedial part of the spring ligament complex of the foot: a study of cadavers and asymptomatic volunteers. Skeletal Radiol 2007;36:221.
32. Deland JT, Lee KT, Sobel M, et al. Anatomy of the plantar plate and its attachments in the lesser metatarsal phalangeal joint. Foot Ankle Int 1995;16:480.
33. Johnston RB 3rd, Smith J, Daniels T. The plantar plate of the lesser toes: an anatomical study in human cadavers. Foot Ankle Int 1994;15:276.
34. Umans HR, Elsinger E. The plantar plate of the lesser metatarsophalangeal joints: potential for injury and role of MR imaging. Magn Reson Imaging Clin N Am 2001; 9:659.
35. Wang B, Guss A, Chalayon O, et al. Deep transverse metatarsal ligament and static stability of lesser metatarsophalangeal joints: a cadaveric study. Foot Ankle Int 2015;36:573.

Fibrocartilaginous Tissue
Why Does It Fail to Heal?

John T. Marcoux, DPM, DABFAS, FACFAS[a],*,
Lowell Tong, DPM, PMSR / RRA PGY-3[b]

KEYWORDS

- Tendon • Ligament • Bone • Interface • Enthesis • Healing • Fibrocartilage

KEY POINTS

- Tendon/ligament to bone interface healing has mixed evidence of success due to its limited regeneration capability.
- Fibrocartilaginous entheses are more prone to injury, and healing at the entheses is not well understood.
- Various intrinsic and extrinsic factors contribute to failed healing.
- Tendon and ligaments heal through 3 consecutive phases with the formation of fibrovascular scar tissue that is mechanically weaker and more prone to failure.
- Advanced biological treatment has shown some promise in augmenting healing but further research is needed to ascertain clinical efficacy.

INTRODUCTION

Tendons and ligaments are critical components in the function of the musculoskeletal system, as they provide stability and guide motion for the biomechanical transmission of forces into bone. Several common injuries in the foot and ankle require the repair of ruptured or attenuated tendon or ligament to its osseous insertion. Understanding the structure and function of injured ligaments and tendons is complicated by the variability and unpredictable nature of their healing. The healing process at the tendon/ligament to bone interface is challenging and often frustrating to foot and ankle surgeons, as they have a high failure rate necessitating the need for revision; this may be due to the dramatic physiologic and structural changes that ligaments and tendons sustain as a result of injury, as well as the complex and dynamic cellular processes that occur during healing. These processes create alterations in the biology and biomechanics of the injured tendon and/or ligament, leading to inadequate healing and tissue formation that is inferior to the tissue it replaces. The primary contributors to less than optimal

[a] Division of Podiatry, Department of Surgery, Beth Israel Deaconess Medical Center, Harvard Medical School, 185 Pilgrim Road, Span 3, Boston, MA 02215, USA; [b] Division of Podiatry, Department of Surgery, Beth Israel Deaconess Medical Center, 185 Pilgrim Road, Span 3, Boston, MA 02215, USA
* Corresponding author.
E-mail address: jmarcou2@bidmc.harvard.edu

Clin Podiatr Med Surg 39 (2022) 437–450
https://doi.org/10.1016/j.cpm.2022.02.005
0891-8422/22/© 2022 Elsevier Inc. All rights reserved.

outcomes have been attributed to poor local blood supply at the insertion site, continued biomechanical or structural deformity, and the limited regenerative capacity at the tendon/ligament to bone interface due to the nature of the tissues and the diverse mechanical properties seen at these areas of high stress.

LIGAMENTS

Ligaments prevent excessive motion of joints by providing stability of the joint at rest and through normal range of motion; this allows ligaments to transfer a tensile load to and from the skeleton while dynamically distributing the loads applied to them in order to perform specific movement patterns.[1] Ligaments also function to provide joint homeostasis through their viscoelastic properties that reflect the complex interactions between collagens, proteoglycans, water, and other proteins.[2,3] The viscoelastic properties, along with the recruitment of crimped collagen, contribute to the mechanical behavior of the ligament under loading conditions. When tension is applied, ligaments deform, or elongate, in a nonlinear fashion through the recruitment of crimped collagen fibers. As the tension placed on the ligament increases, the collagen fibers progressively uncrimp, or elongate, until all fibers are nearly linear.

The ligament structure increasingly stiffens as the ligament fibers are stretched and become increasingly linear. Varying degrees of ligament stiffness are necessary for various loads and various ranges of joint motion. When ligaments are exposed to loading over an extended period of time, they increase in mass, stiffness, and load to failure.[4] When this occurs, the ligament becomes lax and unable to properly support the joint, leading to instability and pain. When an applied load causes all fibers to become nearly linear, the ligament continues to absorb energy until tensile failure or disruption of the tissue.

Overstretched and ligament disruptions/tears lead to joint instability. In an attempt to prevent overstretching and disruption, ligaments exhibit both creep and relaxation behaviors. Creep and load relaxation behaviors help to prevent fatigue failure of the tissue when ligaments are loaded in tension. Creep is defined as the deformation, or elongation, of a ligament over time under a constant load or stress. Load relaxation refers to a decrease in stress of the tissue over time when the ligament is subjected to a constant elongation.[5-7]

When ligaments are overloaded, or exposed to tensions greater than the structures can sustain, they fail, resulting in partial or complete ligament discontinuity. Ligament injuries create disruptions in the balance between joint mobility and joint stability. If healing is inadequate to regain functional static stability, abnormal force transmission continues throughout the joint, resulting in damage to other musculoskeletal structures in and around the joint.

TENDONS

A tendon's primary functional responsibility is to translate the load of muscular contractions to joint movement. The principal role of the tendon is to resist tension; however, they must allow for a certain degree of compliance within musculoskeletal biomechanics. A tendon is stronger per unit area than muscle and has a tensile strength approximately equal to bone but with additional flexibility, elasticity, and extensibility. The parallel arrangement of collagen fibers acts to resist tension so that contractile energy is not lost during load transmission. The loads encountered in everyday activities are typically well below the tissue's ultimate tensile strength; however, in quick eccentric contraction that can occur with rapid deceleration, more significant stresses can be observed, which can result in tendon injury.[8,9]

Tendons are living connective tissue, which consist of dense yet flexible type I collagen fibrils oriented in a parallel fashion embedded in a hydrated proteoglycan matrix. The structure is maintained by tenocytes, which are primarily responsible for maintaining the extracellular matrix in response to its environment. The smallest structural unit is the collagen fibril. Each fibril is built from soluble tropocollagen molecules forming cross-links to create insoluble collagen molecules, which then aggregate progressively into microfibrils, fibrils, and finally fibers. Bundles of fibers are bound together by thin layers of loose connective tissue known as the epi- and endotenon, which allow the fiber groups to glide on each other in an almost frictionless manner. They also carry blood vessels, nerves, and lymphatics to the deeper portions of the tendon. The paratenon in tendons with a straight course or the synovial sheath in tendons with an angled course support the tendon and is composed of a loose, fatty, areolar tissue, or synovial sheath.[10]

This 3-dimensional structure provides the tendon with high tensile force and resilience while preventing separation of the fibers under mechanical stress. In the past, it was generally believed that tendons were avascular with low metabolic activity. We now understand that the tendon derives its blood supply from several main sources. An understanding of this vascular supply is necessary in order to ensure that healing can be observed following injury or surgical repair. Tendons obtain their blood supply from muscular branches at the myotendinous junction, vessels from the mesotenon or paratenon, and lastly vessels at the tendo-osseous junction. The branches from the myotendinous junction only supply the distal or proximal one-third of the tendon, and the mesotenon provides circulation to the entirety of the tendon. There are some areas of compromised vasculature, which is believed to lead to predictably weak areas predisposed to rupture.[11]

Controversy surrounds the pathogenesis of tendinopathy, as it is not fully understood at the current time. There is a multitude of extrinsic and intrinsic factors that may influence the development of tendinopathy.[12] Extrinsic factors include occupation, sporting activities, local environmental conditions, posture, and biomechanical factors. Intrinsic factors include age, gender, body weight, anatomic variation, and systemic diseases such as diabetes mellitus.[13,14]

It is extremely rare for a healthy tendon to develop a spontaneous intrasubstance tendon rupture following rapid, strong tensile loading of the tendon. It would be more likely that one would suffer an avulsion fracture at the tendon insertion site or myofascial injury. Tendons in the foot such as the tibialis posterior, peroneal tendons, and Achilles tendon are much more likely to develop attritional tears based on the biomechanical stresses applied to them. Repetitive eccentric loading of these tendons is implicated as a major cause in the development of progressive tendinopathy and subsequent rupture. Characteristic changes occur in tendon structure that results in a tendon being incapable of sustaining repeated tensile loads. Acute overload within the tendon is sensed by the tenocyte, which results in a cascade of cell-based reactive physiologic responses.[15]

Several models regarding the cause for tendon pathology have been proposed. These have been divided into 3 main categories:

1. Collagen disruption/tearing
2. Inflammation
3. Tendon cell response

Cook and Purdam in 2009 proposed a model of tendon pathology based around a continuum model, which incorporates clinical, histologic, and imaging information. Their model describes the early stages of reactive tendon pathology as a noninflammatory, proliferative tissue reaction, usually in response to acute overload or compression.[16] The tendon thickens due to the upregulation of large proteoglycans and an increase in bound water, with minimal collagen damage or separation. Tendon dysrepair is characterized by greater tissue matrix breakdown, with collagen separation, proliferation of abnormal tenocytes, and some increase in tendon neovascularity. These first 2 stages are considered to have some degree of reversibility if provided an appropriate healing environment. The final stage is degenerative tendinopathy, an essentially irreversible stage, which sees further disruption of collagen, widespread cell death, and extensive ingrowth of neovessels and nerves into the tendon substance. This model of tendinopathy progression helps to provide a framework describing what treatments might be best aligned with the stage of tendinopathy, along with descriptions of the clinical presentation of each stage.[15]

ENTHESES

The interaction between soft and hard anatomic tissues is essential for musculoskeletal motion and normal biomechanical function. The enthesis is a specialized tissue interface, which facilitates the integration between these 2 dissimilar anatomic structures with widely different mechanical properties. Tendons and ligaments are strong in tension as opposed to the bone, which is well suited for compressive loading. The structural and mechanical properties at tendon/ligament to bone interfaces in the foot are a consequence of the mechanical stresses to which they are exposed and most are described as being fibrocartilaginous.

Fibrocartilaginous entheses are more prone to injury from chronic use and consist of 4 distinct zones with varying cell types, extracellular composition, and mechanical functions. Zone 1: *pure dense fibrous connective tissue* is composed primarily of fibroblasts and type 1 collagen with properties similar to midsubstance tendon. Zone 2: *uncalcified fibrocartilage* is a relatively avascular zone made up of fibrochondrocytes, proteoglycan aggrecan, and type 1, 2, and 3 collagen. The function of this zone is to dissipate bending of the collagen fibers in the tendon. The tidemark separates zones 2 and 3 to provide the mechanical boundary between the soft and hard tissues. Zone 3: *calcified fibrocartilage* is an avascular zone of calcified fibrochondrocytes and predominantly type 2 collagen. This zone provides mechanical integrity to the enthesis. Zone 4: *bone* consists of osteoclasts, osteocytes, and osteoblasts residing in a matrix of type 1 collagen and provides the site of attachment of the tendon (**Fig. 1**).

The body's ability to heal at the entheses interface is not well understood. Studies have reported that the zones developed in normal enthesis development are not fully regenerated during the healing process. Healing results in the formation of fibrovascular scar tissue that is mechanically weaker and more prone to failure, especially in these areas that are subject to overuse injuries and repetitive stress.[17]

TENDON/LIGAMENT HEALING

Tendon and ligaments heal through a distinct sequence of cellular and molecular cascades that occur throughout 3 main consecutive phases: acute inflammatory phase, proliferative or regenerative phase, and tissue remodeling phase. Progression through the phases is not standardized between tendons and ligaments, as ligaments are relatively avascular compared with tendons.

The phases of healing overlap, and their duration depends on the location and severity of the damage. The initial phase is the acute inflammatory phase, which begins in the first 48 to 72 hours after injury. The platelet-rich fibrin clot that develops

| tendon
(zone I) | fibrocartilage
(zone II + III) | bone
(zone IV) |

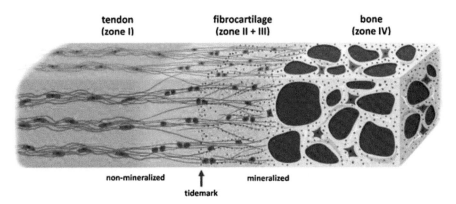

non-mineralized   ↑   mineralized
tidemark

Fig. 1. A direct enthesis with 4 interwoven zones. Histologically, the basic scaffold is based on a largely oriented fiber course of collagens and a corresponding orientation of the cell axes in the tendon zone (I), whereas cartilage and bone zones have less or no such orientation of the fibers. Major differences in the composition result from different cell types, molecules of the extracellular matrix, and mineral content. (*From* Friese N, Gierschner MB, Schadzek P, Roger Y, Hoffmann A. Regeneration of Damaged Tendon-Bone Junctions (Entheses)—TAK1 as a Potential Node Factor. International Journal of Molecular Sciences. 2020; 21(15):5177. https://doi.org/10.3390/ijms21155177).

releases various chemotactic factors, which attract inflammatory cells to the injured area.

This is followed by the reparative or proliferative stage, which starts ~72 hours after the injury and lasts for ~6 weeks. It involves the recruitment of various growth factors and cytokines to provide a vascular network responsible for the survival of newly forming fibrous tissue at the injury site. Fibroblasts are continuously recruited, and proteoglycans, collagens, and other components of the extracellular matrix are synthesized and then arranged randomly within the matrix. The tendon or ligament in this stage appears as disorganized scar tissue and has an extensive blood vessel network.

The remodeling stage is the last phase of healing and is divided into a consolidation and maturation component. The consolidation component of the remodeling stage begins ~6 to 8 weeks following the injury and is characterized by a decrease in cellularity and matrix production, as the tissue becomes more fibrous through the replacement of type III collagen by type I collagen. The collagen fiber structure becomes more organized, which helps to restore stiffness and tensile strength. After ~10 weeks into the healing process, the maturation stage begins and can continue for months to years. This includes an increase in collagen fiber cross-linking and the formation of more normal appearing mature tissues.[9,18–20] Unfortunately, the healing process at the tendon/ligament to bone interface does not achieve the same characteristics and critical differences in matrix structure and function persist (**Table 1**).

In fact, evidence suggests that the injured ligament structure is replaced with tissue that is grossly, histologically, biochemically, and biomechanically similar to scar tissue.[21–24] As Frank and colleagues[2] note, even fully remodeled scar tissue remains grossly, microscopically, and functionally different from normal tissues.

Numerous strategies have been used over the years attempting to improve tendon and ligament healing after injury or surgery. In general, tendons and ligaments are influenced by their mechanical environments. Failure to recognize and address underlying biomechanical or structural deformity results in continued strain and failure of the involved tendon or ligament. In the foot and ankle, biomechanical imbalance related to

Table 1 Phases of tendon/ligament healing		
Inflammatory	The blood vessels within the tendon sheath create the formation of a hematoma. The resulting clot releases various chemotactic factors, which attract inflammatory cells	48–72 h
Repair/proliferative	Recruitment of various growth factors to provide a vascular network responsible for the survival of newly forming fibrous tissue at the injury site	Begins day 3 to 6 wk
Remodeling	Consolidation—characterized by a decrease in cellularity and matrix production. Replacement of type III collagen by type I collagen. The collagen fiber structure is organized along the longitudinal axis of the tendon, which helps to restore tendon stiffness and tensile strength	Begins 6–8 wk postinjury
	Maturation—increase in collagen fiber cross-linking and the formation of more mature tendon tissue	Begins 10 wk postinjury

excessive protonation and equinus often leads to structural deformities such as hallux valgus, hammertoe deformities, rearfoot valgus, and medial column insufficiency. These biomechanical and structural deformities need to be addressed as part of the holistic approach to management; failure to do so often results in failed healing of the tendon and/or ligament and recurrence of deformity, pain, and impaired function.

Once the tendon or ligament has been repaired, early resumption of controlled range of motion can stimulate repair, restoration of function, and avoid adhesions. It is imperative that the repair is solid and gap formation at the healing interface is avoided. The treatment of tendon and ligament injuries with prolonged immobilization may delay recovery and adversely affect tissue maturation and stiffness.

The use of corticosteroids for tendon and ligament injuries is controversial. The mechanism behind any positive effect for their use is unclear. Some believe that any beneficial effect of corticosteroids arises from the suppression of inflammation, which include lyses of tendon adhesions.[25] Corticosteroid injections may have a short-term benefit, but studies demonstrate that the adverse effects of inhibited fibroblast function and subsequent collagen synthesis result in atrophy, decreased tensile strength, and load to failure.[26,27]

Nonsteroidal antiinflammatory drugs (NSAIDs) are commonly used as first-line treatment of tendon and ligament injuries. Their mechanism of action is to inhibit the cyclooxygenase (COX) enzymes in the arachidonic acid (ArA) pathway to reduce synthesis of prostaglandins, which are inducers of inflammation.

Within the ArA cycle there are 2 cyclooxygenase isoforms: COX-1 and COX-2. COX-1 is constitutively expressed in many cell types, whereas COX-2 is inductively expressed. Proinflammatory stimuli including lipopolysaccharide and tumor necrosis factor are potent inducers of COX-2 expression. The prostaglandins produced via COX-1 or COX-2 subsequently amplify or sustain the inflammation response and if inhibited results in a reduction of blood flow to the injury site, which negatively affects fibroblast proliferation.

Corticosteroid injections and nonsteroidal antiinflammatory medications have been shown to be effective in decreasing inflammation and pain; however, the histologic, biochemical, and biomechanical properties of tendon and ligament healing are inhibited. For this reason, their use is cautioned in individuals who have tendon and ligament injuries, as they may increase the risk for spontaneous rupture. As such, NSAIDs are no longer recommended for chronic tendon and ligament injuries and for acute tendon and ligament injuries should be used for the shortest period of time, if used at all.[28]

PLANTAR PLATE

The plantar plate disruption is a common forefoot pathology, which most frequently involves the second metatarsophalangeal joint. It is often associated with hallux abducto valgus deformity and medial column insufficiency, which results in submetatarsal overload. It is an intracapsular, fibrocartilaginous ligament consisting primarily of type 1 collagen. It originates on the plantar metatarsal neck and inserts into the base of the proximal phalanx and measures approximately 20 mm in length, 15 mm in width, and 2 to 5 mm in thickness.[29] It serves as the terminal attachment of the plantar fascia and receives contributions from the intrinsic muscles of the foot, paired collateral ligaments, flexor tendon sheath, and deep transverse intermetatarsal ligaments.

The plantar plate is in direct contact with the metatarsal head and is the primary static stabilizer of the lesser metatarsophalangeal joints in the sagittal plane and cushions axial load on the metatarsal head much as the meniscus in the knee.[29] It resists tensile loads during dorsiflexion and supports the windlass mechanism as the distal insertion of the plantar fascia. Dynamic stability of the lesser metatarsophalangeal joints is provided by the extrinsic and intrinsic musculature. Various anatomic and biomechanical studies have concluded that metatarsophalangeal joint stability depends on the integrity of the plantar plate, and if compromised, dorsal displacement of the proximal phalanx occurs, and the ability of the intrinsic and extrinsic musculature attachments are unable to provide dynamic stability to the lesser metatarsophalangeal joint.[30–33]

Depending on the extent of plantar plate disruption at the metatarsophalangeal joint, the toe may sublux or dislocate in the sagittal plane dorsally with or without transverse plane instability either medially or laterally due to the pull of the intrinsic musculature[30] (**Fig. 2**).

The ability for the plantar plate to heal and regain static stability across the metatarsophalangeal joint once it has been compromised and deformity develops has been a challenge for foot and ankle surgeons. The biological capacity of the plantar plate to

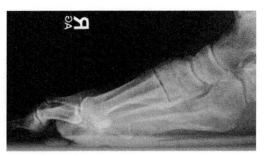

Fig. 2. Lateral weight-bearing radiograph of plantar plate disruption with dorsal subluxation of the second metatarsophalangeal joint.

heal has been implicated as a concern based on the vascular anatomy of this fibrocartilaginous structure. It has been established that a tissue's ability to heal is directly linked to the vascular supply to provide an inflammatory response and nutrition.[34] Recent studies have been conducted to investigate and define the microvascular perfusion of the plantar plate using nano-computerized tomography. Finney and colleagues in their cadaveric study concluded that there was a vascular network extending from the surrounding soft tissues into approximately the proximal 20% to 30% and the distal 20% of the plantar plate. A hypovascular midportion of the plantar plate may play an important role in the underlying pathoanatomy and pathophysiology of the area.[35]

Singer and colleagues performed a follow-up cadaveric study to compare the intact plantar plate microvascular network with the microvascular network of plantar plates in the presence of toe deformity using a similar perfusion and non–computed tomography imaging method. They concluded that torn plantar plates exhibited neovascularization around the site of the plantar plate tear that did not exist in normal plantar plates. In comparison to intact plantar plates, they visualized a more robust vascular network extending from the surrounding soft tissues, which was most notable in the distal attachment areas of the plantar plate. The clinical significance of neovascularization in torn plantar plates is unknown at this time but it suggests that the plantar plate is attempting to heal.[36]

Mann compared the association between metatarsal protrusion distance on foot radiographs with plantar plate tears on MRI. They retrospectively compared 166 patients (211 feet). Anteroposterior and lateral weight-bearing radiographs were obtained as well as forefoot MR images. Radiographic measurements were obtained to determine the relative second metatarsal length. Lines were drawn perpendicular to the apex of the second metatarsal head as well as a line drawn between the distal margins of the first and third metatarsal heads. MRI studies were reviewed, and the plantar plate was classified as normal, completely torn, or partially plantar torn/degenerated. Results demonstrated an association between length of protrusion of the second metatarsal and plantar plate tear. They concluded that a second metatarsal protrusion length of 5 mm was strongly associated with a plantar plate pathology.[37]

SPRING LIGAMENT

Spring ligament complex is the main static support for the medial longitudinal arch. The posterior tibial tendon functions as the primary dynamic stabilizer to support the medial arch. Pathology of the spring ligament and posterior tibial tendon dysfunction is often accompanied by equinus. Failure of these stabilizers results in rearfoot instability, which permits plantarflexion of the talus with the development of pes planovalgus.

The spring ligament complex is composed of 3 distinct components, the superomedial, inferoplantar, and medioplantar calcaneonavicular ligaments. The superomedial calcaneonavicular ligament is a thick fibrocartilaginous band that lies directly medial to posterior tibial tendon and blends into the deltoid complex. The superomedial component provides support for the medial aspect of the talar head and functions as a hammock to maintain the anatomic relationship with the calcaneus and midtarsal joint.[38]

The inferoplantar calcaneonavicular ligament is a small fibrous structure that lies beneath the talonavicular. It takes origin from the coronoid fossa anterior to the medioplantar calcaneonavicular ligament and inserts on the inferior aspect of the navicular tuberosity. The medioplantar calcaneonavicular ligament originates from the coronoid fossa at the anterior aspect of the calcaneus and inserts beneath the tuberosity of the navicular.[39]

The calcaneonavicular ligament complex was originally thought to act as a spring for the longitudinal arch of the foot but histologic and biomechanical analysis of the ligament reveals that it is purely collagenous and has no elastic properties.[40]

Assessment of the spring ligament complex reveals that the superomedial part of the spring ligament complex is usually affected. Assessment of the superomedial calcaneonavicular ligament in study groups with posterior tibial tendinosis and an asymptomatic control group revealed a mean proximal thickness of 4 mm and a distal thickness of 3.6 mm in the control group. The posterior tibial tendinopathy group had statistically significant difference in thickness with a mean proximal measurement of 5.1 mm ($P < .01$) and a distal thickness of 6.1 mm ($P < .001$)[41] (**Fig. 3**).

It is necessary that the foot and ankle surgeon addresses the structural deformity and biomechanical faults in an attempt to restore the spring ligament ability to provide static support to the medial column. Acevedo and Vora used an "internal brace" augmentation of the spring ligament with a fiber tape construct on 26 patients. The augmentation was performed in combination with various additional procedures for flatfoot reconstruction including flexor digitorum longus transfer with posterior tibial tendon debridement with or without side-to-side anastomosis, medial calcaneal displacement osteotomy, gastrocnemius recession, and other procedures as needed. The investigators concluded that the efficacy in studying any one procedure in flatfoot surgery is difficult; however, the spring ligament internal brace augmentation in combination with other osseous and soft tissue procedures was found to be reproducible and demonstrated a more stable construct with dramatic improvement in talonavicular uncoverage and medial column sag.[42]

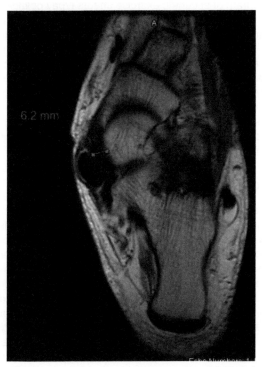

Fig. 3. MRI image of a 61-year-old woman with posterior tibial tendon dysfunction and spring ligament thickening greater than 5 mm.

A study by Kelly and colleagues demonstrated diminished tibiotalar static joint reactive force in a spring ligament injury. They noted subsequent joint reactive force restoration using two-limbed reconstruction of the deltoid and spring ligament using a semitendinosis allograft to reconstruct the tibionavicular and tibiocalcaneal ligaments in a cadaveric model.[43]

INSERTIONAL ACHILLES TENDINOPATHY

Insertional Achilles tendinopathy management is difficult with many treatment approaches advocated in the literature; this is often an overuse injury that occurs in athletes such as distance runners, skiing, skating, and those involved in jumping sports. The Achilles tendon is the strongest tendon in the body; it originates from the soleus muscle with 2 muscle bellies of the gastrocnemius, and the tendon inserts distally onto the posterior, central aspect of the calcaneus. Blood supply to the tendon comes from 3 different sources: muscle-tendon junction, tendon-bone junction, and the length of the tendon from the sheath. That central portion is vascularized by the surrounding paratenon. The least vascularized portion, known as the watershed area is approximately 2 to 6 cm above the insertion.

One may see a retrocalcaneal traction exostosis with or without tendon calcification or prominence of the posterosuperior aspect of the calcaneus (**Fig. 4**). There is a consensus that conservative options such as stretching and eccentric exercises in physical therapy should be exhausted before proceeding with surgical intervention. Eccentric exercise alters tendon pathology in both the short term and the long term. In the short term, a single bout of exercise increases tendon volume and signal intensity on MRI.[44] A program of eccentric exercise affects type I collagen production and, in the absence of ongoing insult, may increase the tendon volume over the longer term.[45] As such, an eccentric exercise program may increase tensile strength in the tendon over time. The effect of repetitive stretching, with a "lengthening" of the muscle–tendon unit, may also have an impact on capacity of the musculotendinous unit to effectively absorb load.[46]

If surgical intervention becomes necessary, adequate debridement of diseased tendon and resection of intratendinous calcification and remodeling of the retrocalcaneal exostosis should be performed. The tendon should be reattached with a stable tendon anchoring construct that will allow early controlled range of motion to prevent adhesions and stimulate repair at the tendon to bone interface.

EMERGING TECHNOLOGIES

Advanced biological treatments for tendon and ligament pathology have gained popularity in the literature to augment the healing process. Plate-rich plasma (PRP) is an autologous, highly concentrated platelet blood product that is obtained by centrifuging venous blood to remove red blood cells. PRP contains several cytokines and proteins that act as cell adhesion molecules and growth factors. These growth factors include 3 isomers of platelet-derived growth factors (PDGFaa, PDGFbb, and PDGFab), 2 of the numerous transforming growth factors (TGF1 and TGF2), vascular endothelial growth factor, and epithelial growth factor.[47] Because this is an autologous product, there is variability in the growth factors that are present in PRP. The evidence regarding PRP continues to evolve in tendon and ligament pathology but there is a lack of unbiased clinical outcome studies. One significant drawback to widespread clinical use is a high out-of-pocket expense to the patient, as this treatment is rarely covered by insurance.

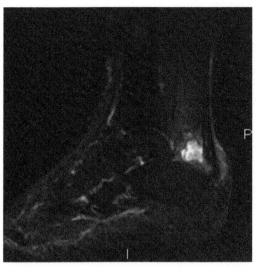

Fig. 4. Intraoperative picture demonstrating chronic insertional tendinopathy with tendon degeneration.

Mesenchymal stem cells (MSC) therapy is another emerging biological treatment. MSCs are typically harvested from autologous fat or bone marrow and have the ability to differentiate into multiple tissue types including tenocytes, chondrocytes, osteoblasts, and myoblasts, which theoretically would allow regeneration of the tendon to bone interface. Many growth factors and molecules contained in PRP are produced and released by MSCs in response to a tissue injury. Recent studies have shown that MSCs rarely make a direct contribution to tissue regeneration but indirectly stimulate tissue repair by secreting trophic factors, which activate residual recipient cells and/or modulate the inflammatory response.[48–52]

The use of these emerging technologies is encouraging; there remains a lack of understanding in how these biological approaches can be best used to promote tendon and ligament healing. Further research to the overall efficacy is still needed; however, it remains a viable conservative treatment with low risk of complications and adverse reactions.

SUMMARY

Tendon/ligament to bone healing in the foot and ankle continues to be a challenge and often frustrates patients and clinicians. The structure and function of injured ligaments and tendons are complicated by the variability and unpredictable nature of their healing. Less than optimal outcomes have been attributed to avascularity at the insertion site, biomechanical or structural deformity, and the limited regenerative capacity at the tendon/ligament to bone interface due to the nature of the tissues and the diverse mechanical properties seen at these areas of high stress. Although conservative and surgical approaches continue to evolve, healing unfortunately results in the formation of fibrovascular scar tissue that is mechanically weaker and more prone to failure, especially in the foot and ankle, which is subject to overuse injuries and repetitive stress.

CLINICS CARE POINTS

- Biomechanical and structural deformities need to be addressed as part of the holistic approach to management; failure to do so often results in failed healing of the tendon and/or ligament and recurrence of deformity, pain, and impaired function.

- Once the tendon or ligament has been repaired, early resumption of controlled range of motion can stimulate repair, restoration of function, and avoid adhesions.

- Corticosteroid injections and nonsteroidal antiinflammatory medications have been shown to be effective in decreasing inflammation and pain; however, the histologic, biochemical, and biomechanical properties of tendon and ligament healing are inhibited.

- For this reason, their use is cautioned in individuals who have tendon and ligament injuries, as they may increase the risk for spontaneous rupture.

DISCLOSURE

The authors have nothing to disclose.

REFERENCES

1. Benjamin M, Toumi H, Ralphs JR, et al. Where tendons and ligaments meet bone: attachment sites ('entheses') in relation to exercise and/or mechanical load. J Anat 2006;208(4):471–90.
2. Frank CB. Ligament structure, physiology and function. J Musculoskelet Neuronal Interact 2004;4(2):199–201.
3. Jung HJ, Fisher MB, Woo SL. Role of biomechanics in the understanding of normal, injured, and healing ligaments and tendons. Sports Med Arthrosc Rehabil Ther Technol 2009;1(1):9.
4. Vereeke WK, Fu F. Soft-tissue physiology and repair. In: Vaccaro A, editor. Orthopaedic knowledge update 8. Rosemont (IL): American Academy of Orthopaedic Surgeons; 2005. p. 15–27.
5. Frank C, Shrive N, Bray R, et al. Ligament healing a review of some current clinical and experimental concepts. Iowa Orthop J 1992;12:21–8.
6. Akeson WH, Frank CB, Amiel D, et al. Ligament biology and biomechanics. In: Finerman G, editor. American academy of orthopaedic surgeons symposium on sports medicine: the knee. St Louis (MO): CV Mosby Co; 1985. p. 111.
7. Andriacchi TP, DeHaven KE, Dahners LE, et al. Ligament injury and repair. In: Woo SL-Y, Buckwalter JA, editors. Injury and repair of the musculoskeletal soft tissues. Park Ridge (IL): Am Acad Orthop Surg; 1988. p. 103.
8. James R, Kesturu G, Balian G, et al. Tendon: biology, biomechanics, repair, growth factors, and evolving treatment options. J Hand Surg Am 2008;33(1): 102–12.
9. Lin TW, Cardenas L, Soslowsky LJ. Biomechanics of tendon injury and repair. J Biomech 2004;37(6):865–77.
10. Gagliano N, Menon A, Martinelli C, et al. Tendon structure and extracellular matrix components are affected by spasticity in cerebral palsy patients. Muscles Ligaments Tendons J 2013;3(1):42–50.
11. Fenwick SA, Hazleman BL, Riley GP, et al. The vasculature and its role in the damaged and healing tendon. Arthritis Res 2002;4(4):252–60.
12. Lewis JS. Rotatorcufftendinopathy:amodelforthecontinuumofpathologyandrelated management. Br J Sports Med 2010;44:918–23.

13. DeOliveira RR, Lemos A, De Castro Silveira PV, et al. Alterations of tendons in patients with diabetes mellitus: a systematic review. Diabet Med 2011;28:886–95.

14. Gaida JE, Alfredson H, etal. AsymptomaticAchillestendonpathologyassociated-withacen- tral fat distribution in men and peripheral fat distribution in women: a cross-sectional study of 298 individuals. BMC Musculoskelet Disord 2010;11:41.

15. Cook JL, Rio E, Purdam CR, et al. Revisiting the continuum model of tendon pathol- ogy: what is its merit in clinical practice and research? Br J Sports Med 2016;50:1187–91.

16. Cook JL, Purdam CR. Is tendon pathology a continuum? A pathology model to explain the clinical presentation of load-induced tendinopathy. Br J Sports Med 2009;43(6):409–16.

17. Apostolakos J, Durant TJS, Dwyer CR, et al. The enthesis: a review of the tendon-to-bone insertion. Muscles Ligaments Tendons J 2019;4(3):333.

18. Docheva D, Müller SA, Majewski M, et al. Biologics for tendon repair. Adv Drug Deliv Rev 2015;84:222–39.

19. Yang G, Rothrauff BB, Tuan RS, et al. Tendon and ligament regeneration and repair: clinical relevance and developmental paradigm. Birth Defects Res C Embryo Today 2013;99(3):203–22.

20. Galloway MT, Lalley AL, Shearn JT. The role of mechanical loading in tendon development, mainte- nance, injury, and repair. J Bone Joint Surg Am 2013; 95(17):1620–8.

21. Shepherd JH, Screen HR. Fatigue loading of tendon. Int J Exp Pathol 2013;94(4): 260–70.

22. Tang JB, Zhang Y, Cao Y, et al. Core suture purchase affects strength of tendon repairs. J Hand Surg Am 2005;30(6):1262–6.

23. Wu YF, Tang JB. Recent developments in flexor tendon repair techniques and factors influencing strength of the tendon repair. J Hand Surg Eur 2014; 39(1):6–19.

24. Cheung Y, Rosenberg ZS, Magee T, et al. Normal anatomy and pathologic conditions of ankle tendons: current imaging techniques. Radiographics 1992;12(3): 429–44.

25. Magnussen RA, Dunn WR, Thomson AB. Nonoperative treatment of midportion Achilles tendinopathy: a systematic review. Clin J Sport Med 2009;19(1):54–64.

26. Nichols AW. Complications associated with the use of corticosteroids in the treatment of athletic injuries. Clin J Sport Med 2005;15(5):370–5.

27. Li H-Y, Hua Y-H. Achilles TENDINOPATHY: current concepts about the basic science and clinical treatments. Biomed Res Int 2016;2016:1–9.

28. Su B, O'Connor JP. NSAID therapy effects on healing of bone, tendon, and the enthesis. J Appl Physiol (1985) 2013;115(6):892–9.

29. Johnston RB 3rd, Smith J, Daniels T. The plantar plate of the lesser toes: an anatomical study in human cadavers. Foot Ankle Int 1994;15(5):276–82.

30. Nery C, Lemos AVKC, Raduan F, et al. Combined spring and deltoid ligament repair in adult-acquired flatfoot. Foot Ankle Int 2018;39(8):903–7.

31. Flint WW, Macias DM, Jastifer JR, et al. Plantar plate repair for lesser metatarsophalangeal joint instability. Foot Ankle Int 2017;38(3):234–42.

32. Doty JF, Coughlin MJ. Metatarsophalangeal joint instability of the lesser toes. J Foot Ankle Surg 2014;53(4):440–5.

33. Yu GV, Judge MS, Hudson JR, et al. Predislocation syndrome. Progressive subluxation/dislocation of the lesser metatarsophalangeal joint. J Am Podiatr Med Assoc 2002;92(4):182–99.

34. Bray RC, Rangayyan RM, Frank CB. Normal and healing ligament vascularity: a quantitative histological assessment in the adult rabbit medial collateral ligament. J Anat 1996;188(Pt 1):87–95.

35. Finney FT, McPheters A, Singer NV, et al. Microvasculature of the plantar plate using nano-computed tomography. Foot Ankle Int 2019;40(4):457–64.

36. Singer NV, Saunders NE, Holmes JR, et al. Presence of neovascularization in torn plantar plates of the lesser metatarsophalangeal joints. Foot Ankle Int 2021;42(7): 944–51.

37. Mann TS, Nery C, Baumfeld D, et al. Is second metatarsal protrusion related to metatarsophalangeal plantar plate rupture? AJR Am J Roentgenol 2021;216(1): 132–40.

38. Taniguchi A, Tanaka Y, Takakura Y, et al. Anatomy of the spring ligament. J Bone Joint Surg Am 2003;85(11):2174–8.

39. Rule J, Yao L, Seeger LL. Spring ligament of the ankle: normal MR anatomy. AJR Am J Roentgenol 1993;161(6):1241–4.

40. Davis WH, Sobel M, DiCarlo EF, et al. Gross, histological, and microvascular anatomy and biomechanical testing of the spring ligament complex. Foot Ankle Int 1996;17(2):95–102.

41. Mansour R, Teh J, Sharp RJ, et al. Ultrasound assessment of the spring ligament complex. Eur Radiol 2008;18(11):2670–5.

42. Acevedo J, Vora A. Anatomical reconstruction of the spring LIGAMENT COMPLEX. Foot Ankle Spec 2013;6(6):441–5.

43. Kelly M, Masqoodi N, Vasconcellos D, et al. Spring ligament tear decreases static stability of the ankle joint. Clin Biomech (Bristol, Avon) 2019;61:79–83.

44. Shalabi A, Kristoffersen-Wiberg M, Aspelin P, et al. Immediate Achilles tendon response after strength training evaluated by MRI. Med Sci Sports Exerc 2004; 36(11):1841–6.

45. Kjaer M, Langberg H, Miller BF, et al. Metabolic activity and collagen turnover in human tendon in response to physical activity. J Musculoskelet Neuronal Interact 2005;5(1):41–52.

46. Alfredson H, Cook J. A treatment algorithm for MANAGING Achilles TENDINOPATHY: new treatment options. Br J Sports Med 2007;41(4):211–6.

47. Riel H, Lindstrøm CF, Rathleff MS, et al. Prevalence and incidence rate of lower-extremity tendinopathies in a Danish general practice: a registry-based study. BMC Musculoskelet Disord 2019;20(1):239.

48. Aggarwal S, Pittenger MF. Human mesenchymal stem cells modulate allogeneic immune cell responses. Blood 2005;105(4):1815–22.

49. Caplan AI. Why are MSCs therapeutic? new data: new insight. J Pathol 2009; 217(2):318–24.

50. Rees JD, Pilcher J, Heron C, et al. A comparison of clinical vs ultrasound determined synovitis in rheumatoid arthritis utilizing gray-scale, power Doppler and the intravenous microbubble contrast agent 'Sono-Vue'. Rheumatology (Oxford) 2007;46(3):454–9.

51. Schu S, Nosov M, O'Flynn L, et al. Immunogenicity of allogeneic mesenchymal stem cells. J Cell Mol Med 2012;16(9):2094–103.

52. Youngstrom DW, LaDow JE, Barrett JG. Tenogenesis of bone marrow-, adipose-, and tendon-derived stem cells in a dynamic bioreactor. Connect Tissue Res 2016;57(6):454–65.

Nonoperative Treatment of Plantar Plate Tears

Karan Malani, DPM, Madison Ravine, DPM, Harry P. Schneider, DPM*

KEYWORDS

- Fibrocartilage • Hammertoe • Lesser metatarsophalangeal joint • Plantar plate
- Predislocation syndrome

KEY POINTS

- The plantar plate is a principal static stabilizer of the metatarsophalangeal joint, which when disrupted, allows for the development and progression of digital deformity.
- Conservative treatment is most efficacious on patients who are in the early stages of the deformity.
- Reports of conservative treatment modalities in the literature are largely limited to case studies and series.
- Based on the pathophysiology of the plantar plate, conservative treatment will not allow for anatomic repair of the fibrocartilaginous structure.

INTRODUCTION

The differential diagnoses for forefoot pain, specifically localized metatarsophalangeal joint (MTPJ) pain, are rather broad and encompass principally musculoskeletal and neurologic causes. Among the musculoskeletal causes considered, plantar plate pathology remains one of the most commonly encountered. Although various treatment modalities for plantar plate pathology exist, most literature discusses operative management, and as such, there is a paucity of data regarding nonoperative treatment. Furthermore, both operative and nonoperative treatments of plantar plate pathology are accompanied by inconsistent outcomes and notable challenges to both patient and physician. The purpose of the following article is to further detail the cause of plantar plate insufficiency, focusing on conservative treatment options, outcomes, and limitations.

CAUSE OF PLANTAR PLATE INSUFFICIENCY

The plantar plate is a fibrocartilaginous intraarticular structure serving as one of the primary static stabilizers of the metatarsophalangeal joints. It is predominantly

Cambridge Health Alliance, 1493 Cambridge Street, Department of Surgery, Cambridge, MA 02139, USA
* Corresponding author.
E-mail address: hschneider@challiance.org

Clin Podiatr Med Surg 39 (2022) 451–459
https://doi.org/10.1016/j.cpm.2022.02.006
0891-8422/22/© 2022 Elsevier Inc. All rights reserved.
podiatric.theclinics.com

composed of collagen type 1, with fibers coursing in a manner designed to resist tension and withstand compression.[1–4] Distally, it attaches to the plantar base of the proximal phalanx, and this represents its weakest point. Plantar plate pathology is most commonly seen at the second MTPJ; however, it can be seen at the third and fourth MTPJs as well. A 2012 prospective study by Nery and colleagues[5] revealed that the demographics of plantar plate pathology involve the second MTPJ in 64% of cases, third MTPJ in 32% of cases, and fourth MTPJ in 4% of cases.

Certainly, plantar plate tear or rupture can be acute in presentation, as the result of an acute trauma; this will typically present with pain rather than deformity.[1,6] More often, however, the pathology is chronic and progressive in nature. With this chronic presentation, patients may present with edema and pain in the early stages, progressing to cross-over toe, hammer toe, and floating toe deformity in the later stages. The MTPJ stability provided by the plantar plate is principally static in nature. During the propulsion and toe-off phases of gait, the proximal phalanx is forcefully dorsiflexed on the MTPJ. Resisting this ground reactive force is the plantar plate, which functions with the intrinsic musculature and collateral ligaments to maintain the proximal phalanx in a neutral position. As pathology develops in the plantar plate, beginning with thickening and attenuation, culminating in partial tear or complete rupture, this static stabilizer is lost; this leads to deformity in the sagittal plane: dorsal subluxation or dislocation at the MTPJ. The lumbrical tendons, however, remain intact and insert onto the medial aspect of the extensor hood apparatus. These exert an adductory force at the MTPJ, resulting in a medial deviation of the digit and subsequent deformity in the transverse plane.[3,6] As the flexor tendons continue to exert their force across the joint, this leads to further contracture and eventual hammertoe deformity.[6] Over time, the remaining static structures of the intrinsics and collateral ligaments will also attenuate and no longer be able to compensate for the lost plantar plate, worsening the degree of deformity seen in late stages. Furthermore, certain anatomic factors such as elongated second metatarsal, hallux valgus deformity, first ray hypermobility, pes planus, and equinus deformity may lead to increased load-bearing on the lesser MTPJs, predisposing the patient to develop the aforementioned.[1,2,6]

CLINICAL EVALUATION AND PERTINENT FINDINGS

Patients presenting with plantar plate pathology typically endorse pain and inflammation localized to the plantar aspect of the digital sulcus, just distal to the metatarsal head along the base of the proximal phalanx.[1,2,6] Pain is typically present with propulsion during gait as well as with activity and can be reproduced with direct palpation. Patients may oftentimes endorse localized edema as well. They may endorse neuritic symptoms complicating diagnosis; however, there should be no pain with medial to lateral compression across the transverse metatarsal arch with plantar plate pathology; this may present as a chief complaint of feeling they are "walking on a marble."[6,7] That being said, it is important to note that this may be the typical presenting symptom in the early stage of pathology; however, deformity may be the chief complaint in later stages.

In terms of physical examination findings, in a non–weight-bearing attitude, one may observe any degree of deformity including contracture of the MTPJ and/or proximal interphalangeal joint, cross-over toe, and digital subluxation or dislocation. When the foot is loaded, there may be an exacerbation of symptoms including medial deviation or splaying of the digits and dorsal dislocation. On transition to weight-bearing, this may translate as a lack of digital purchase. Certain specific testing may be performed including a Modified Lachman's test or dorsal excursion, which will elicit pain, guarding, or deficit.[1,2] The Modified Lachman's test, also referred to as the drawer test in certain texts, is strikingly sensitive and specific for lesser MTPJ instability, with a reported 80.6% sensitivity and 99.8% specificity.[8] In addition, associated findings such as hallux valgus deformity, first ray hypermobility, or insufficiency may be appreciated. Differential diagnoses considered at this point include intermetatarsal neuroma, metatarsal stress fracture, capsulitis, osteoarthritis versus inflammatory arthritis, crystalline or infectious arthropathy, or Frieberg infraction to name a few.[1]

The first line of imaging generally obtained for plantar plate pathology includes a standard 3-view weight-bearing radiograph series. On the anteroposterior projection, one may assess for deviation of the digit at the MTPJ in the transverse plane, digital deformity, hallux valgus deformity, metatarsal length patterns, and anatomic parabola. On the lateral projection, one may evaluate the degree of digital deformity in the sagittal plane, specifically evaluating for possible dorsal dislocation of the metatarsophalangeal and interphalangeal joints, as well as assess for elevation of the first ray or first ray hypermobility.[1,2,6] The oblique projection may further be used to assess the alignment of the MTPJ, as well as the presence or absence of intraarticular degenerative changes. Although plain films allow for assessment of the biomechanical and structural evidence and sequelae of plantar plate pathology, advanced imaging such as MRI or ultrasound is required to visualize the plantar plate itself. MRI may be obtained following plain films and allows for direct visualization of effusion, thickening, attenuation, partial tear, or complete rupture of the plantar plate. The thickness of the plantar plate, which is typically 2 to 3 mm, may be increased to 4 to 6 mm in the setting of pathology.[1] It should be noted, however, that inherent limitations to MRI exist, which lead to false positives and false negatives. That being said, MRI does provide utility in that it allows for ruling out other differential diagnoses mentioned earlier.[2] Less frequently, musculoskeletal ultrasound and diagnostic arthrography may also be used with excellent effect to assess the plantar plate in a more dynamic fashion.[1,6,9] Although ultrasound utility is generally limited by technician-dependent factors, it may be more sensitive than MRI, whereas MRI is more specific.[8]

CONSERVATIVE TREATMENT OF PLANTAR PLATE TEARS

There are a variety of nonoperative treatment options used in the management of plantar plate pathology; however, their overall efficacy is debated with no clear protocol established. In addition, the scarce literature available regarding conservative management requires patients to adhere to a long, cumbersome treatment plan. As a result, patient education is a highly important part of the treatment where clinicians should provide information regarding the disease process, treatment plan, the importance of compliance, and potential for surgical intervention.[10]

Conservative treatment is usually only performed on patients who are in the early stages of the deformity or grades 0 to 2 on the Coughlin grading (**Table 1**).[10] Unfortunately, because of the insidious nature of the deformity and the slow progression of symptoms, patients usually only seek treatment once the deformity has progressed to a Coughlin grade 3 or higher.[8] Even though conservative therapy may help alleviate pain, it cannot eliminate symptoms or correct the underlying deformity. Nonsteroidal antiinflammatory medications are usually the first line of treatment of acute inflammation, but these rarely relieve all symptoms.[8] In the acute phase, offloading and immobilization can also be attempted. Use of a postoperative shoe can provide the appropriate symptomatic relief. One can also add a soft insole to further help reduce the stress to the plantar aspect of the forefoot. Alternatively, application of a metatarsal pad proximal to the site of the symptoms can aid in redistributing weight along

Table 1
Clinical staging system for metatarsophalangeal joint instability

Grade	Alignment	Physical Examination
0	MTPJ aligned; prodromal phase with pain, without deformity	MTPJ pain and swelling, reduced toe purchase, negative drawer sign
1	Mild malalignment of MTPJ; widening of web space, medial deviation of digit	MTPJ pain and swelling, loss of toe purchase, mild positive drawer (< 50% subluxable)
2	Moderate malalignment; medial, lateral, dorsal or dorsomedial deformity, hyperextension of digit	MTPJ pain, reduced swelling, loss of toe purchase, moderate positive drawer (> 50% subluxable)
3	Severe malalignment; dorsal or dorsomedial deformity; second toe can overlap hallux; may have flexible hammertoe	MTPJ and toe pain, mild swelling, no toe purchase, very positive positive drawer (dislocatable MTPJ), flexible hammertoe
4	Dorsomedial or dorsal dislocation; severe deformity with dislocation; fixed hammertoe	MTPJ and toe pain, little to no swelling, no toe purchase, dislocated MTPJ, fixed hammertoe

Adapted from Coughlin MJ, Baumfeld DS, Nery C. Second MTP Joint Instability: Grading of the Deformity and Description of Surgical Repair of Capsular Insufficiency. Phys Sportsmed 2011;39(3):132-41.[12]

the forefoot, thus reducing stress to the affected digit.[8] One should ideally complement appropriate offloading with splinting and joint stabilization as well.[10,11] Taping the affected digit in a 10° plantarflexed position will reduce sagittal plane instability, help further reduce pain, and lead to fibrosis of the torn plantar plate, as demonstrated in **Fig. 1**.[8,10] Clinicians should be wary of the risks of taping, however, as it can lead to edema and ulcerations.[7,8,10] In such situations, a Budin splint can be an excellent alternative.[10] Silicone toe sleeves can help relieve pain as well; however, these are more directed toward pain associated with hammertoes that develop secondary to plantar plate ruptures; this is demonstrated in **Fig. 2**. Intraarticular corticosteroid injections have also been reported in literature to be used for symptomatic pain relief. However, these must be used judiciously, as repeat injections can lead to further degeneration and attenuation of the already damaged plantar plate[8,10,12]; This can subsequently result in subluxation and ultimately dislocation of the digit. If an injection is performed, the digit should be stabilized externally through buddy taping or splinting.[10,13] Prolotherapy injections have also been attempted with positive outcomes published in literature, but should be complemented by physical therapy, offloading shoes, and stabilization of the affected digit through taping or splinting.[14] Patients involved in athletic activities should also be instructed to suspend all weight-bearing athletic activities until symptoms have significantly improved and the Modified Lachman is negative.[10,11]

There does not seem to be any level 1 or level 2 evidence demonstrating the efficacy of conservative therapy for plantar plate pathology. However, individual case studies detailing its success exist in literature. Jordan and colleagues published a case report of a 48-year-old female recreational athlete with a plantar plate rupture at the second MTPJ approximately 6 months after suffering a water-skiing accident. Patient was treated conservatively with a regimen of taping of the second digit in 10° of plantarflexion combined with a forefoot unloading shoe and a selective cushioning insole for the second MTPJ. The tape was secured in a crossed fashion starting dorsally at the proximal end of the digit and extended plantarly and crossing at the ball of the foot with the

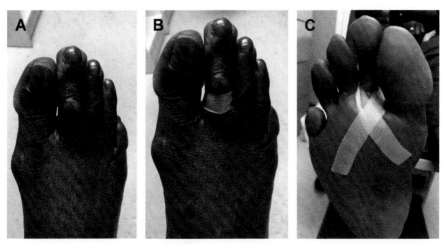

Fig. 1. (A) Second digit with plantar plate pathology. (B) Dorsal view of taping. (C) Plantar view of taping.

digit held in 10° plantarflexion. The patient was trained in the taping technique and was instructed to wear the shoe full time. She was followed-up at 3, 6, 8, and 12 months with MRI scans taken at 3, 8, and 12 months. The patient did not demonstrate significant improvement after 3 months of treatment. However, significant clinical signs of improvement were noted at 6 months posttreatment. After 1 year of treatment, the patient had returned to all previous activity without any pain or limitation. The patient's 1-year MRI scans also showed full healing of the plantar plate.[11] Ojofeitimi and colleagues published a similar case report of a 33-year-old female professional dancer who was seen with a 2-week history of second and third MTP joint soreness and pain in the demi pointe position. Physical examination and imaging studies demonstrated second MTPJ capsulitis and plantar plate rupture with concomitant plantar fasciitis. The plantar fasciitis resolved after 7 weeks of physical therapy. However, the patient's second MTPJ pain remained despite buddy taping, use of antiinflammatories, and supportive conservative therapy consisting of rest, ice, compression, elevation. The patient continued to dance during this time. As a result, the patient was ultimately placed in a postoperative shoe with a Budin splint maintaining the digit in a neutral position. After demonstrating minimal improvement despite 3 weeks of treatment, the patient was ultimately given prolotherapy injections consisting of a series of 4 injections. Each injection consisted of 1 mL of 25% dextrose and 0.5% lidocaine. The injections were spread over 16 weeks with the first 2 injections 2 weeks apart. The patient was also initiated on a 3-phase rehabilitation program, which included strengthening, posture improvement, and retraining of dance technique to allow appropriate weight distribution across the forefoot. After 37 physical therapy sessions over 6 weeks and 4 prolotherapy sessions in total, the patient was able to perform all dance choreography with taping and padding; however, he still demonstrated continued difficulty with turning and jumping activities on the affected side. It took the patient an additional year before being able to dance pain free without taping or padding.[14]

Both of the aforementioned case reports demonstrate successful outcomes for both acute and chronic tears; however, the length of treatment can last upward of 1 year and can be quite challenging for the patient. The therapies that might be effective for each individual patient may also vary depending on baseline activity level and

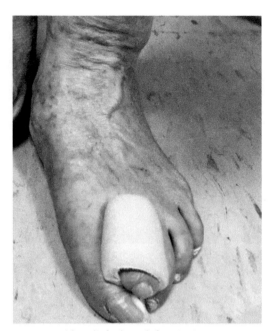

Fig. 2. Digital sleeve may provide relief when deformity is present.

demand. Future studies with a larger patient population will definitely help create a more defined nonoperative treatment protocol for management of plantar plate ruptures.

PATTERN OF PLANTAR PLATE TEARS AND EFFECT ON CONSERVATIVE MANAGEMENT

Coughlin and colleagues[15] developed an anatomic grading system describing the pattern of plantar plate tears ranging from plantar plate attenuation and/or discoloration (grade 0) to an extensive tear with button hole and a combination of transverse and longitudinal tear (grade 4) (**Fig. 3**, **Table 2**). Naturally, more extensive tears correlate with more substantial angular digital deformity and worse clinical symptoms, including increased pain, swelling, positive Modified Lachman test, and chronicity of symptoms. The higher graded plantar plate tears are less likely to respond to conservative therapy; however, the authors are unaware of any studies to date that assess conservative versus surgical treatment based on the type of tear. This area has an extensive scope for further research and could be quite beneficial for both patients and practitioners.

LIMITS OF CONSERVATIVE TREATMENT

Based on a review of the literature, the authors were unable to find any published studies regarding the conservative treatment of plantar plate ruptures, except for the aforementioned cases studies. There are no randomized controlled studies, nor are there published case series regarding conservative treatment. Based on the pathophysiology of the plantar plate, conservative treatment will not allow anatomic repair of the fibrocartilaginous structure. In grade 0 tears, taping or splinting in early stages

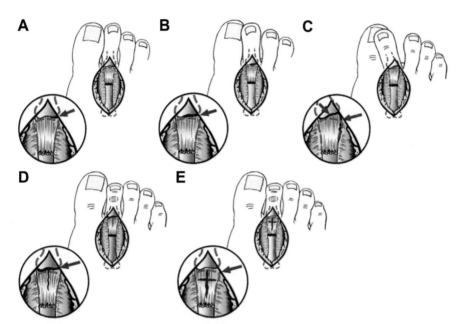

Fig. 3. Anatomical grading of plantar plate tears: (A) grade 1 tear, (B) grade 2 tear, (C) grade 3 tear, (D) grade 3 tear (another type), and (E) grade 4 (arrows denote tears). (Reprinted with permission from Surgery of the Foot and Ankle, 9th ed, Figures 7-84.) (*From* 8. Doty J, Coughlin M, Jastifer J, Weil L Jr, Nery C. Evaluation and Treatment of Lesser Metatarsophalangeal Joint Instability: The Repair of Plantar Plate Insufficiency Through a Dorsal Approach. Oper Tech Sports Med 2014;22:339-47).

may prevent worsening of the pathology and will mitigate pain. In later stages, taping may help relieve pain but will not correct the deformity. Randomized controlled trials of taping/splinting would be beneficial to understand the true limitations of conservative treatment.

SUMMARY

The differential diagnosis for patients presenting with forefoot pain are broad and diverse; however, plantar plate pathology should be strongly considered and remain at the forefront of the clinician's mind. The plantar plate is a vital structure involved

Table 2 Pattern of plantar plate tears	
Grade	Pattern of Plantar Plate Tear
0	Plantar plate attenuation, discoloration, degeneration
1	Transverse distal tear (<50%) (adjacent to insertion at distal phalanx)
2	Transverse distal tear (>50%) (adjacent to insertion at distal phalanx)
3	Transverse and longitudinal extensive tear (may involve the collateral ligaments)
4	Extensive tear with little plantar plate present (usually an irreparable tear)

Adapted from Doty JF, Coughlin MJ, Weil L Jr, Nery C. Etiology and Management of Lesser Toe Metatarsophalangeal Joint Instability. Foot Ankle Clin N Am 2014;19:358-405.[6]

in maintaining stability across the metatarsophalangeal joints during stance and gait alike. Its disruption, either through acute trauma or chronic repetitive wear and tear, can not only be painful for the patient but may also lead to subsequent secondary structural deformities. Symptoms associated with plantar plate ruptures are quite insidious in nature. Hence, a thorough physical examination and appropriate use of imaging are essential to helping a clinician formulate their diagnosis. There are several conservative therapy options available to help alleviate symptoms associated with plantar plate ruptures. These range from splinting to offloading in postsurgical shoes to administration of corticosteroid injections. Unfortunately, once the pathology progresses to the more advanced stages, the efficacy of these treatment options becomes compromised. Success with nonoperative treatment has been demonstrated in isolated case reports where patients presented in the early stages of the deformity. However, reports are limited to low-level evidence. As such, there is a clear need for additional research in this area to not only evaluate the true efficacy of conservative therapies but also to help devise a standardized approach for the overall management of plantar plate pathology.

CLINICS CARE POINTS

- Plantar plate pathology may be either acute or chronic in nature and leads to painful digital deformity.
- Reports of conservative treatment modalities for plantar plate pathology are limited to low-level clinical evidence.
- Conservative treatment modalities are most beneficial in the earlier stages of pathology and may prevent worsening of the pathology and mitigate pain.

DISCLOSURE

H.P. Schneider is a consultant and speaker for Smith & Nephew. The other authors have nothing to disclose.

REFERENCES

1. Camasta CA. Chapter 19: plantar plate repair of the second metatarsophalangeal joint. McGlammary's comprehensive textbook of foot and ankle surgery. 4th edition. Lippincott Williams & Wilkins; 2012. p. 187–201.
2. Bavarian B, Thompson J, Nazarian D. Plantar plate tears: a review of the modified flexor tendon transfer repair for stabilization. Clin Podiatr Med Surg 2011;28: 57–68.
3. Nery C, Umans H, Baumfeld D. Etiology, clinical assessment, and surgical repair of plantar plate tears. Semin Musculoskelet Radiol 2016;20(2):205–13.
4. Deland JT, Lee KT, Sobel M, et al. Anatomy of the plantar plate and its attachments in the lesser metatarsal phalangeal joint. Foot Ankle Int 1995;16(8):480–6.
5. Nery C, Coughlin MJ, Baumfeld D, et al. Lesser metatarsophalangeal joint instability: prospective evaluation and repair of plantar plate and capsular insufficiency. Foot Ankle Int 2012;33(4):301–11.
6. Doty JF, Coughlin MJ, Weil L Jr, et al. Etiology and management of lesser toe metatarsophalangeal joint instability. Foot Ankle Clin N Am 2014;19:358–405.
7. Coughlin MJ. Subluxation and dislocation of the second metatarsophalangeal joint. Orthop Clin North Am 1989;20(4):535–51.

8. Doty J, Coughlin M, Jastifer J, et al. Evaluation and treatment of lesser metatar-sophalangeal joint instability: the repair of plantar plate insufficiency through a dorsal approach. Oper Tech Sports Med 2014;22:339–47.

9. Blitz NM, Ford LA, Christensen JC. Second metatarsophalangeal joint arthrogra-phy: a cadaveric correlation study. J Foot Ankle Surg 2004;43(4):231–40.

10. Kitner CW, Hodgkins CW. Lesser Metatarsophalangeal instability: diagnosis and conservative management of a common cause of metatarsalgia. Sports Health 2020;12(4):390–4.

11. Jordan M, Thomas M, Fischer W. Nonoperative treatment of a lesser toe plantar plate tear with serial MRI follow-up: a case report. J Foot Ankle Surg 2017;56: 857–61.

12. Coughlin MJ, Baumfeld DS, Nery C. Second MTP joint instability: grading of the deformity and description of surgical repair of capsular insufficiency. Phys Sportsmed 2011;39(3):132–41.

13. Smith BW, Coughlin MJ. Disorders of the lesser toes. Sports Med Arthrosc Rev 2009;17(3):167–74.

14. Ojofeitimi S, Bronner S, Becica L. Conservative management of second metatar-sophalangeal joint instability in a professional dancer: a case report. J Orthop Sports Phys Ther 2016;46(2):114–23.

15. Coughlin MJ, Schutt SA, Hirose CB, et al. Metatarsophalangeal joint pathology in crossover second toe deformity: a cadaveric study. Foot Ankle Int 2012;33(2): 133–40.

Injuries to the Spring Ligament
Nonoperative Treatment

Douglas H. Richie Jr, FACFAS, DPM*

KEYWORDS

- Posterior tibial tendon dysfunction • PTTD • Adult acquired flatfoot deformity
- AAFD • Progressive collapsing flatfoot deformity • PCFD • Ankle-foot orthoses

KEY POINTS

- The spring ligament can rupture in isolation or accompanying rupture of the posterior tibial tendon
- The spring ligament is the key supportive structure of the talocalcaneonavicular articulation
- Rupture of the spring ligament is a pivotal event in the progressive collapsing foot deformity (PCFD).
- Bracing the PCFD must address hindfoot eversion, forefoot inversion, collapse of the medial longitudinal arch, and forefoot abduction
- Studies of nonoperative treatment of the PCFD using ankle-foot orthoses and focused rehabilitation show favorable results in most patients treated.

INTRODUCTION

The spring ligament can be ruptured in isolation or may be injured in combination with the posterior tibial tendon as well as other key ligaments of the medial ankle and hindfoot.[1,2] Isolated spring ligament injuries are rarely reported and more often considered part of the global condition now known as the progressive collapsing foot deformity (PCFD).[3] Previously, the PCFD was described as posterior tibial tendon dysfunction (PTTD) or the adult acquired flatfoot deformity (AAFD). Both terms have been used in previous published research, which are cited in this article.

The critical stage in the development of the PCFD is rupture of the spring ligament.[3] Once spring ligament injury is detected, the patient has already suffered profound and progressive change in foot alignment with potential for significant long-term disability.[4]

California School of Podiatric Medicine at Samuel Merritt University, 450 30th Street Suite 2860, Oakland, CA 94609, USA
* Corresponding author.
E-mail address: drichiejr@aol.com

Clin Podiatr Med Surg 39 (2022) 461–476
https://doi.org/10.1016/j.cpm.2022.02.007   **podiatric.theclinics.com**

This finding underscores the crucial role played by the spring ligament in maintaining the unique biomechanical function of the human foot.

This article focuses on the role of the spring ligament in PCFD. The pathoanatomy and pathomechanics of spring ligament injuries are explored. Based on this knowledge, a protocol for nonoperative management of spring ligament injuries is proposed.

ANATOMY

Historically, the term "spring ligament" has been assigned to various ligaments connecting the calcaneus and the navicular.[5,6] However, isolated spring ligament injury is attributed to the superomedial calcaneonavicular (SMCN) ligament connecting the middle facet of the sustentaculum of the calcaneus to the superior, medial, and inferior borders of the navicular articular cartilage[1] (**Fig. 1**). Davis and coworkers[7] published a detailed description of the SMCN ligament and the entire "spring ligament complex." Key to the findings of the study by Davis and colleagues[7] was the recognition of an anatomic connection between the SMCN and inferior calcaneonavicular ligaments as well as the posterior tibial tendon and the superficial deltoid ligament.

After the study by Davis and colleagues,[7] several investigators verified the close anatomic and functional relationship between the deltoid ligament of the ankle and the spring ligament complex. Cromeens and colleagues[8] found that the combined medial collateral (deltoid) and spring ligament complexes were composed of multidirectional bands of tissue connecting 4 different bones and spanning 3 synovial joints. The articulation of the SMCN ligament with the head of the talus has fibrocartilage and was thus described by Cromeens and colleagues[8] as a "glenoid" structure. Amaha and coworkers[9] also observed that the medial collateral ligaments of the ankle blend with and become part of the spring ligament complex.[9]

The articulations spanned by the spring ligament complex include the ankle, subtalar, and talonavicular joints. These joints do not function independent of each other because their movements are all kinematically coupled.[10] What is clear is that the combined talocalcaneonavicular joint is the critical articulation of the adult acquired flatfoot (AAF)[11,12]; this dispels a long-held belief that the pathomechanics of the disorder originates primarily at the subtalar joint.[13–15]

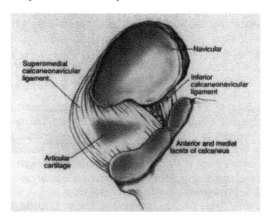

Fig. 1. The superomedial calcaneonavicular ligament. (*From* Davis WH, Sobel M, DiCarlo EF, et al. Gross, histological, and microvascular anatomy and biomechanical testing of the spring ligament complex. Foot Ankle Int. 1996;17(2):Figure 4 p. 97. This also appeared in: Richie DH. Biomechanics and clinical analysis of the adult acquired flatfoot. Clin Podiatr Med Surg 2007;24:617-44 as Figure 1, page 623.)

The talonavicular joint is the most mobile of all the joints in the human foot during ambulation.[10] Compared with the calcaneocuboid joint, the talonavicular joint lacks any type of intrinsic osseous features to provide anatomic "locking" for stability. Instead, the talonavicular joint relies on an intricate complex of ligaments for stability. MacConaill[16] draws an analogy between the talonavicular joint and the hip joint. In this classic article, MacConaill[16] refers to the hip joint as the "acetabulum coxae," whereas the talonavicular joint is described as the "acetabulum pedis." Unlike the hip, however, MacConaill[16] observed that the talonavicular joint was a hinged structure in the transverse plane, pivoting laterally and constrained by the medial sling of the bifurcate ligament and the SMCN ligament. The term "acetabulum pedis" has been adopted by several anatomists describing the spring ligament complex and the talocalcaneonavicular joint[17,18] (**Fig. 2**).

PATHOANATOMY AND PATHOMECHANICS OF SPRING LIGAMENT INJURY

Davis and colleagues[7] found that the tensile strength of the SMCN ligament was less than body weight and is of comparable strength to the lateral ankle ligaments. The investigators also observed from histologic studies that the SMCN ligament has a structural arrangement of fibers aligned to resist both tensile and compressive forces. The fibrocartilaginous plate within the spring ligament resists compressive forces from the head of the talus. These compressive forces result from internal rotation of the tibiotalar unit—a motion that is coupled with rearfoot protonation.[16] The SMCN ligament provides the primary medial constraint to adduction or internal rotation of the talus at the talocalcaneonavicular joint.[19] Of important relevance, microvasculature studies by Davis and colleagues[7] showed that the fibrocartilage or articular portion of the SMCN ligament is essentially avascular.

The avascularity of the central part of the superomedial portion of the spring ligament could be a predisposing factor for ligament injury and failure to heal. Also, the native fibrocartilaginous origin of this ligament may lead to progressive attenuation and degeneration from compressive loads resulting from adduction and plantarflexion of the head of the talus.[20,21] Patients who develop rupture of the posterior tibial tendon and subsequent rupture of the spring ligament usually have a preexisting flatfoot deformity.[10–13] Persistent valgus positioning of the hindfoot, coupled with internal

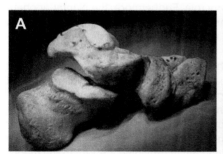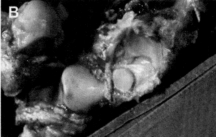

Fig. 2. The articulation and acetabulum of the talocalcaneonavicular joint. (*A*) The talus, navicular, along with the anterior and middle facet of the calcaneus are one distinct articulation known as the talocalcan joint. (*B*) The anterior and middle facet (sustentaculum) of the calcaneus is clearly part of the acetabulum pedis, whereas the posterior facet of the calcaneus is a separate joint. (*From* Pisani G. "Coxa pedis" today. Foot Ankle Surg. 2016 Jun;22(2):78-84. https://doi.org/10.1016/j.fas.2015.05.004. Epub 2015 Jun 23. PMID: 27301725.)

rotation of the tibiotalar unit, increases compression and tensile loads on the spring ligament complex setting up potential for eventual structural failure.[7,10]

The spring ligament can be ruptured in isolation without involvement of the posterior tibial tendon.[22–27] Studies of patients with an isolated rupture of the spring ligament suggest that the injury can have either an acute or a chronic presentation.[22,23] The acute rupture is seen in younger athletic patients who experience an eversion ankle sprain.[24–27] Chronic spring ligament tears are attributed to repetitive stress from compression of the talus, similar to the cause of PTTD or the AAF.[22] Investigators of 2 different reports of chronic isolated rupture of the spring ligament have concluded that this is a different condition than PTTD or the AAF simply because the posterior tibial tendon was still intact.[22,23] However, it is now recognized that spring ligament injury can precede posterior tibial tendon rupture and this ligament injury is the inciting event leading to the AAD.[2–4]

Clinical reports of patients who have suffered attenuation or rupture of the spring ligament consistently describe an acquired progressive deformity of the patient's affected foot characterized by hindfoot eversion, forefoot abduction, and collapse of the medial longitudinal arch.[22–27] This same multilevel deformity has been reported in patients who have suffered rupture of the posterior tibial tendon.[12–14,28] These early reports describing a progressive flatfoot deformity characterized by hindfoot eversion and forefoot abduction attributed the structural changes to loss of function of the posterior tibial tendon alone.[29,30] Subsequent studies have dispelled that notion and verified that the primary event leading to the classic appearance of the AAF is rupture of the spring ligament.

Jennings and Christensen[31] discovered the critical role of the spring ligament in providing stability to the talocalaneaonavicular joint. In this landmark study, the investigators sectioned the SMCN (spring) ligament in 5 cadaveric specimens and applied axial load to the tibia while also loading the posterior tibial tendon. When the spring ligament was sectioned, a significant change of alignment of the medial arch along with calcaneal eversion occurred, which the posterior tibial tendon was unable to compensate.

A more recent study using finite analysis computer modeling to measure stress in key soft tissue structures in stage 2 AAFD confirmed the critical role of the spring ligament.[32] The plantar aponeurosis and the spring ligament were identified to be the 2 primary structures that maintained integrity of the medial longitudinal arch, whereas the posterior tibial tendon played a secondary role. Furthermore, the plantar aponeurosis shows a primary role in preventing arch elongation. The spring ligament was found to have a dual function of controlling motion at the talonavicular joint and subtalar joint.

MacDonald and coworkers[33] evaluated the effects of progressive sectioning of the spring ligament in 9 cadaver specimens placed under physiologic loading. Isolated spring ligament sectioning demonstrated significant changes in alignment of the hindfoot and ankle.[33] The talus was noted to undergo significant adduction and plantarflexion when the spring ligament was sectioned. Also, the tibiotalar and subtalar joints underwent significant valgus rotation after spring ligament sectioning, which demonstrates the global role of the spring ligament in providing stability to the medial arch, the hindfoot, and the ankle.

Pasapula and colleagues[34–36] carried out cadaver and clinical studies showing a link between spring ligament insufficiency and plantar fasciitis as well as instability of the first ray. Pasapula and colleagues[34–36] make a convincing argument that attenuation of the spring ligament is the primary inciting event of the AAFD and have proposed a new classification system of this condition based on spring ligament integrity.[37] The investigators note the large body of evidence showing that spring ligament rupture is an essential part of the progressive AAF deformity and suggest that attenuation of this ligament actually precedes the tenosynovitis seen in the TP tendon in early-stage AAFD. Furthermore, Pasapula and colleagues[34–36] propose that progressive collapse of the longitudinal arch of the foot will not occur with isolated spring ligament failure, but instead is a result of acquired instability of the first metatarsocuneiform joint. The investigators observed that protonation of the hindfoot is resisted by a stable first ray. However, with spring ligament failure, the resultant talonavicular joint instability will cause retrograde hindfoot valgus deformity, which will progressively increase ground reaction forces on the first ray. The stabilizing structures of the first ray will eventually fail, causing dorsiflexion of the medial column upon weight-bearing.[38] Dorsiflexion of the medial column relative to the lateral column will result in a "supination deformity" of the forefoot.

Rupture of the spring ligament has now been recognized as a pivotal event in the progression of the flexible AAFD.[2,4,31,38] Recently a panel of experts evaluated the terminology and previous classification systems for the AAF.[3] The experts recognized the shortcoming of previous staging and classification of deformity, which were based solely on the function of the posterior tibial tendon. As a result, this expert panel concluded:

> However, the anatomy of the flexible AAFD includes far more than a rupture of the PTT, most importantly the spring and deltoid ligaments, specifically the articular support provided by the sling effect of the spring ligament to the TN joint, which must be evaluated and always be taken into consideration when evaluating any AAFD. The relevance of the spring ligament has been neglected with respect to descriptive terminology and not included in classification systems over the decades.

This consensus group recommended renaming the AAFD the PCFD, which involves a complex 3D deformity including hindfoot valgus, forefoot abduction, and midfoot supination. Although midfoot supination is a result of medial arch flattening, the panel chose to abandon the term "flatfoot" in the new nomenclature recognizing that many people with flat feet are asymptomatic.[3]

Notwithstanding, whether in isolation or in combination with other key structures of the arch, hindfoot, and ankle, the spring ligament injury is associated with significant changes in alignment of the foot, which must be addressed in both operative and nonoperative treatment protocols. These treatment protocols use interventions that have already shown efficacy in the treatment of the AAF, now known as the PCFD.

TREATING THE SPRING LIGAMENT INJURY: NONOPERATIVE APPROACH
Efficacy of Nonoperative Treatment of the Spring Ligament Injury

Reports of nonoperative treatment of the isolated spring ligament rupture in the absence of posterior tibial tendon pathology reveal conflicting results. In a study by Tryfonidis and coworkers,[22] 6 of 9 patients avoided surgery when treated with "orthoses," although no description of the devices was provided in the article. In a more recent case series published by Masaragian and coworkers,[1] all 10 patients failed to respond to conservative treatment, which was described as immobilization, ice, longitudinal arch support, and rearfoot varus wedges.

Similarly, Orr and Nunley[23] reported that all 6 of their patients with isolated rupture of the spring ligament failed to respond with conservative treatment, which was described as a combination of orthotic use, immobilization, or activity modification. Again, the description of the orthotic was not provided in this report.

In terms of spring ligament injury combined with posterior tibial tendon rupture, there are numerous reports of positive outcomes of conservative treatment.[39–47] These studies of conservative treatment focus on a global condition described by the investigators as either PTTD or the AAF, but are relevant to this discussion because those same conditions are essentially synonymous with chronic spring ligament injury; this is verified by studies that show that the spring ligament is ruptured or attenuated in 80% to 90% of patients with stage 2 PTTD or AAF.[2,48]

Kulig and coworkers[39] reported significant reduction of pain in patients with stage 1 and stage 2 PTTD using foot orthoses along an innovative rehabilitation program. Chao and colleagues[40] used a custom university of california biomechanics laboratory (UCBL)-type foot orthosis to treat stage 2 AAF and achieved excellent/good results in 70% of the patients. Custom foot orthoses seem to be effective and the intervention of choice when ligaments are intact, as seen in stage 1 and early stage 2 AAF deformities. Prefabricated foot orthoses show no effect on improving alignment of AAF.[41,42]

In clinical studies of stage 2 AAF, a variety of ankle-foot orthoses (AFOs) have achieved notable success in allowing patients to return to activity and avoid surgery. Augustin and colleagues[43] prospectively studied 12 patients with stage 2 PTTD as well as 5 patients with stage 3 PTTD treated with a short custom-molded gauntlet-style AFO. Despite a short follow-up period (mean, 12 months), they found significant improvement in american orthopedic foot and ankle society (AOFAS), foot function index (FFI), and short form (SF)-36 scores. All but 2 patients reported at least moderate improvement in pain and function.

Alvarez and colleagues[44] studied 47 consecutive patients with stage 1 or 2 PTTD in a nonoperative protocol combining orthoses with a structured rehabilitation program. A short articulated AFO was used if symptoms were present for greater than 3 months and a three-quarter-length foot orthosis used if they were present less than 3 months. The median treatment period was 129 days with a minimum follow-up of 1 year. Among the subjects, 89% were subjectively satisfied with their treatment, whereas 80.5% were successful in avoiding surgery and staying brace free during day-to-day activities.

Lin and colleagues[45] used a double metal upright AFO to treat stage 2 AAF in 32 patients. This study had an impressive follow-up of 8.6 years where 79% of the patients remained brace free and had avoided surgery. Overall, 94% of the patients were satisfied or partially satisfied. The researchers concluded that bracing has a "high likelihood" of avoiding surgery in patients with AAF.

Neilson and coworkers used a short articulated custom AFO to treat 64 patients with stage 2 AAF.[47] With this brace, combined with physical therapy, 87.5% of the patients were able to avoid surgery over a 27-month observational period. The authors concluded: *"Our interpretation of these findings is that bracing is, in general, a critical element of satisfactorily alleviating the symptoms of AAFD related to PTTD, and that use of the low articulating AFO may be particularly helpful because it combines a foot orthosis with support of the ankle, while enabling full weight-bearing ambulation."*

These reports verify that a significant percentage of patients who have suffered injury to the spring ligament and are in the early stages of AAF will recover in terms of elimination of symptoms and discontinuation of supportive bracing. A conclusion can be drawn that the spring ligament can heal in a similar fashion to the lateral collateral ligaments of the ankle.[49]

Others share this observation of potential healing of the spring ligament complex.[20,50] It should be noted that although studies using bracing to treat the AAF show impressive results, actual healing of the spring ligament has not been documented with imaging or intraoperative confirmation.

A rehabilitation program can augment brace intervention for the treatment of spring ligament injuries. Kulig and coworkers[51] demonstrated the value of foot orthoses to stimulate activity of the tibialis posterior muscle during the performance of eccentric exercise. The investigators implemented this intervention along with proximal hip strengthening exercises and showed significant improvements in pain and function after a 12-week rehabilitation program.[39]

IMPLEMENTING A NONOPERATIVE TREATMENT PROGRAM FOR SPRING LIGAMENT INJURY
Examination

Attenuation and rupture of the spring ligament will lead to changes in foot alignment, which can be detected in static stance and during gait. In most cases the symptomatic PCFD will present unilateral, so comparison with the unaffected foot will show asymmetry that can be attributed to spring ligament rupture.[52]

Of all the 3D changes in foot alignment that result from spring ligament rupture, transverse plane abduction of the forefoot across the midfoot joints is most evident.[4,28,37] This finding is demonstrated in static stance by the "too many toes sign" visualized from a posterior view[13] (**Fig. 3**). Other less noticeable changes in static foot alignment are lowering of the medial longitudinal arch as well as eversion of the hindfoot.[10,11]

During gait, the foot with spring ligament insufficiency will show increased magnitude of forefoot abduction as well as hindfoot eversion[26,53] (see **Fig. 3**). In addition, excessive midfoot mobility in the sagittal plane will be observed after spring ligament injury.[54] This loss of sagittal plane stability of the midfoot joints will manifest in difficulty or inability of the patient to perform the single-foot heel rise test[11] (**Fig. 4**). Patients with isolated rupture of the spring ligament have difficulty performing this test, and when other ligaments of the medial column are ruptured, the heel rise cannot be performed.[35,52]

Detection of forefoot supination or "supinatus" deformity should be carried out on the patient in both weight-bearing and non-weight-bearing condition (**Fig. 5**). Acquired supination deformity is the result of compensatory motion of the forefoot induced by

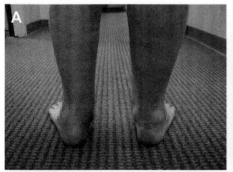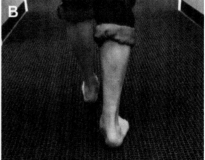

Fig. 3. Forefoot abduction in static stance and during gait. (*A*) Static stance: valgus alignment of the rearfoot along with forefoot abduction, that is, "too many toes," is the result of spring ligament rupture on the left foot. (*B*) During gait, patients with spring ligament rupture show forefoot abduction on the affected side along with delayed heel rise due to midfoot instability.

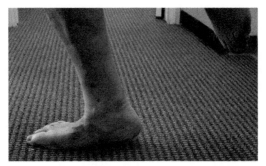

Fig. 4. Inability to complete the single-foot heel rise is due to spring ligament deficiency causing unstable midfoot joints.

eversion of the rearfoot as originally described by Steindler.[55] Persistent valgus collapse of the rearfoot during weight-bearing overloads the medial column causing ligament attenuation.[38] The magnitude, location, and flexibility of forefoot rotation is an important part of staging of the PCFD.[56]

A simple clinical test for spring ligament insufficiency was described by Passapula and colleagues[34] (**Fig. 6**). This "neutral heel lateral push test" has been validated for its direct relevance to spring ligament rupture in 21 cadaver specimens. The test is performed as follows.

The examiner positions the patient's ankle joint in full dorsiflexion and the subtalar joint in a neutral or slightly supinated position. Using the palm of one hand, the examiner stabilizes the lateral aspect of the calcaneus. With the other hand, the examiner applies a lateral force against the medial aspect of the distal first metatarsal. The forefoot is pushed laterally until a firm end point is reached. Comparison is made with the contralateral foot for total transverse plane excursion of the forefoot. A lack of firm end point may also suggest spring ligament rupture.

IMAGING

Rupture of the spring ligament causes significant 3D rotation of joints of the rearfoot and midfoot, which can be measured on weight-bearing radiographs and compared with the contralateral asymptomatic foot.

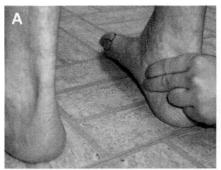
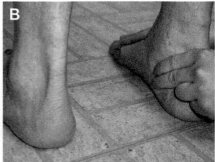

Fig. 5. Acquired forefoot supination deformity detected in weight-bearing examination. (*A*) When the hindfoot corrected to neutral, the forefoot is inverted off the floor. (*B*) Forefoot supination deformity is reducible in stage II adult acquired flatfoot.

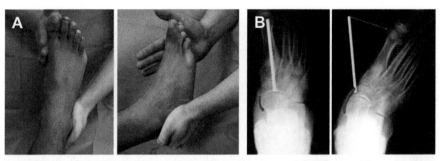

Fig. 6. (*A*) Photographs of the neutral heel lateral push test. (*B*) Radiographic confirmation of neutral heel lateral push causing subluxation of the talonavicular joint. (*Courtesy of Chandra Pasapula, M.D.*)

On the anteroposterior view, forefoot abduction will be evident with increased talonavicular angle and increased uncoverage of the head of the talus.[57] On the standing lateral radiograph, there will be a decrease in calcaneal pitch angle, increased Meary angle (measuring alignment of the medial arch), and decreased height of the distance between the medial cuneiform and the fifth metatarsal[58,59] (**Fig. 7**).

Other imaging studies are not recommended if clinical examination and plain radiographs demonstrate deformity consistent with spring ligament injury. Although MRI can detect the extent of injury ranging from thickening with intrasubstance tears to full-thickness gap, the prognosis for success with nonoperative treatment does not depend on these studies.[48,60]

ORTHOSIS PRESCRIPTION FOR SPRING LIGAMENT INJURY

Foot orthoses have shown efficacy in treating spring ligament injury associated with the AAF,[39,40] whereas AFOs have demonstrated superior effects on controlling the 3D rotation of the talocalcaneonavicular articulation[61–64]; this is explained by the fact that control of internal rotation of the talus at the talonavicular joint is best achieved by control of tibial rotation[64] (**Fig. 8**). Functioning as an intercalary bone without any muscular attachments, the talus is firmly housed within the ankle joint mortise and is directly influenced by tibial rotation.[16,65] Thus, the long lever arm of the tibia can be controlled with an AFO to directly control rotation of the talus (**Fig. 9**).

Studies show that custom molded AFOs correct the deformity associated with the AAF better than prefabricated orthoses.[61,62] Besides custom molding to support the anatomy of the leg, ankle, and foot the impression casting procedure for fabrication of the AFO can be modified to improve control of the complex PCFD. During the

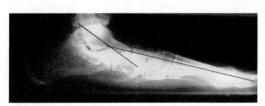

Fig. 7. Rupture of the spring ligament causes loss of sagittal plane stability of the medial column reflected in increased Meary angle on lateral radiograph.

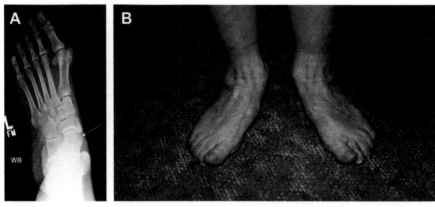

Fig. 8. Radiographic and clinical confirmation of spring ligament rupture. (*A*) Spring ligament rupture causes excessive transverse plane rotation at the talonavicular articulation with uncoverage of the head of the talus. (*B*) Spring ligament rupture causes excessive internal rotation of the tibiofibulotalar unit, clearly visible with clinical inspection of the patient's right foot and comparison with contralateral foot.

impression casting procedure for the custom AFOs, specifically reduction of forefoot supination deformity during the casting procedure is important to produce a device that will reduce rearfoot protonation and reduce strain in the medial column[16,38] (**Fig. 10**).

The positive cast model can be modified to create a medial wedge effect to control protonation of the rearfoot and midfoot. Carlson and Berglund[66] described a method to remove plaster from the plantar aspect of the positive cast beginning at the medial calcaneal tubercle and extending to the sustentaculum area of the positive cast. The end result of this "medial skive" modification of the positive cast is a varus wedge incorporated into the hindfoot portion of the footplate of the brace to provide inversion moment to the subtalar joint (**Fig. 11**). Greater contour to the sustentaculum can enhance support to the talonavicular joint and reduce strain on the SMCN ligament.

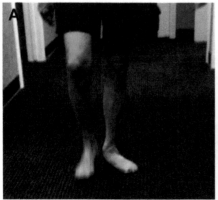
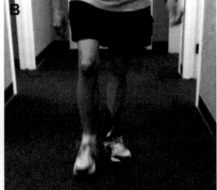

Fig. 9. Ankle-foot orthosis controls internal tibial rotation coupled with forefoot abduction resulting from spring ligament rupture. (*A*) Excessive forefoot abduction. (*B*) Reduction of forefoot abduction via control of internal tibial rotation.

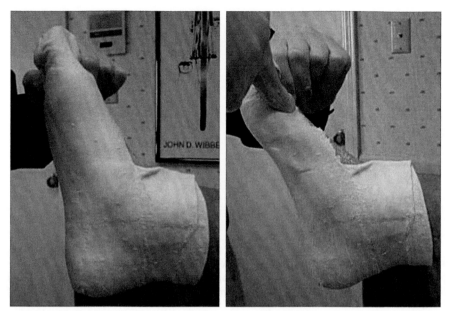

Fig. 10. Reducing forefoot supination deformity in the orthosis impression casting procedure: plantarflexing the medial column.

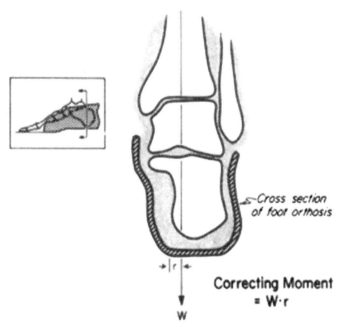

Cross section of foot orthosis

Correcting Moment
= W·r

Fig. 11. Medial skive of positive cast as described by Carlson. (From Carlson JM, Berglund G. An effective orthotic design for controlling the unstable subtalar joint. Orthotics and Prosthetics 1979; 33:1; 39-49. Available at: http://www.oandplibrary.org/op/1979_01_039.asp.)

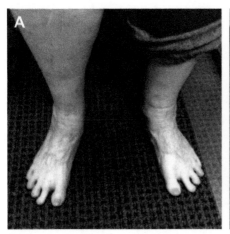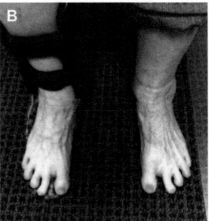

Fig. 12. Spring ligament rupture causing transverse plane instability across the talonavicular joint. (*A*) Asymmetry of forefoot alignment comparing affected right foot with unaffected left foot. (*B*) Forefoot abduction corrected with ankle-foot orthosis and lateral flange of footplate.

Control of forefoot abduction is a key strategy to reducing strain in the spring ligament with orthotic therapy. Neville and colleagues[67] modified a solid AFO with an extension of the lateral wall of the footplateending just proximal to the fifth metatarsophalangeal joint. With this extended "lateral flange," the solid AFO resisted all forefoot abduction, and actually induced slight adduction motion of the forefoot (**Fig. 12**).

CLINICS CARE POINTS

Clinical studies of patients treated conservatively for PTTD/AAF associated with chronic spring ligament injury provide a framework for prognosis:

- Symptoms can be expected to improve within several months of implementation of AFOs.[43,44]
- In those patients who have significant reduction of pain, 50% can expect to be able to discontinue bracing and remain symptom free while wearing foot orthoses and proper footwear.[45,47]
- Patient age, compliance, comorbidities, and extent of deformity can all affect the prognosis for a successful outcome.[43–47]
- There have been no published reports of nonoperative treatment of the spring ligament injury that included treatment with orthobiologics. These interventions offer significant promise to augment the repair of fibrocartilage and should be considered in future studies of spring ligament injury.[68]

SUMMARY

Injury to the SMCN ligament component of the spring ligament complex can result from an acute eversion ankle sprain or from chronic compression of the talus against the fibrocartilaginous portion. Whether acute or chronic, spring ligament injury induces structural change in the alignment of the foot characterized by hindfoot eversion, collapse of the medial longitudinal arch, forefoot supination, and forefoot abduction. Clinical studies show positive outcomes when AFOs are used to specifically address the 3D structural changes in foot alignment induced by spring ligament injury.

DISCLOSURE

D.H. Richie Jr is the owner of Richie Technologies Inc, a company that distributes ankle-foot orthoses.

REFERENCES

1. Masaragian HJ, Massetti S, Perin F, et al. Flatfoot deformity due to isolated spring ligament injury. J Foot Ankle Surg 2020;59:469–78.
2. Deland JT, de Asla RJ, Sung IH, et al. Posterior tibial tendon insufficiency: which ligaments are involved? Foot Ankle Int 2005;26(6):427–35.
3. Myerson MS, Thordarson DB, Johnson JE, et al. Classification and nomenclature: progressive collapsing foot deformity. Foot Ankle Int 2020;41(10):1271–6.
4. Deland JT. Spring ligament complex and flatfoot deformity: curse or blessing? Foot Ankle Int 2012;33(3):239–43.
5. Smith EB. The astragalo-calcaneo-navicular joint. J Anat Physiol 1896;30:238.
6. Hardy RH. Observations on the structure and properties of the plantar calcaneo-navicular ligament in man. J Anat 1951;85:135–9.
7. Davis WH, Sobel M, DiCarlo EF, et al. Gross, histological, and microvascular anatomy and biomechanical testing of the spring ligament complex. Foot Ankle Int 1996;17(2):95–102.
8. Cromeens BP, Kirchhoff CA, Patterson RM, et al. An attachment-based description of the medial collateral and spring ligament complexes. Foot Ankle Int 2015; 36:710–21.
9. Amaha K, Nimura A, Yamaguchi R, et al. Anatomic study of the medial side of the ankle base on the joint capsule: an alternative description of the deltoid and spring ligament. J Exp Orthopaedics 2019;6(2):2–9.
10. Nester CJ, Jarvis HL, Jones RK, et al. Movement of the human foot in 100 pain free individuals aged 18–45: implications for understanding normal foot function. J Foot Ankle Res 2014;7:51.
11. Deland JT, Arnoczky SP, Thompson FM. Adult acquired flatfoot deformity at the talonavicular joint: reconstruction of the spring ligament in an in vitro model. Foot Ankle Int 1992;13:327–32.
12. Nair P, Deland J, Ellis SJ. Current concepts in adult acquired flatfoot deformity. Curr Orthopaedic Pract 2015;26(2):160±8.
13. Mann RA, Specht LH. Posterior tibial tendon ruptures and analysis of eight cases. Foot Ankle 1982;2:350.
14. Mann RA, Thompson FM. Rupture of the posterior tibial tendon causing flatfoot. J Bone Joint Surg 1985;67A:556–61.
15. Mueller TJ. Ruptures and lacerations of the tibialis posterior tendon. J Am Podiatry Assoc 1984;109–19.
16. MacConaill MA. The postural mechanism of the human foot. Proc R Irish Acad 1945;50B:265–78.
17. Vadell AM, Peratta M. Calcaneonavicular ligament: anatomy, diagnosis, and treatment. Foot Ankle Clin 2012;17(3):437–48.
18. Pisani G. Coxa pedis today. Foot Ankle Surg 2016;22:78–84.

19. Reeck J, Felten N, McCormack AP, et al. Support of the talus: a biomechanical investigation of the contributions of the talonavicular and talocalcaneal joints, and the superomedial calcaneonavicular ligament. Foot Ankle Int 1998;19(10): 674–82.

20. Domzalski M, Kwapisz A, Zabierek S. Morphology of spring ligament fibrocartilage complex lesions. J Am Podiatr Med Assoc 2019;109(5):1–5.

21. Benjamin M, Ralphs JR. Fibrocartilage in tendons and ligaments - an adaptation to compressive load. J Anat 1998;193(4):481–94.

22. Tryfonidis M, Jackson W, Mansour R, et al. Acquired adult flat foot due to isolated plantar calcaneonavicular (spring) ligament insufficiency with normal tibialis posterior tendon. Foot Ankle Surg 2008;14:89–95.

23. Orr JD, Nunley JA. Isolated spring ligament failure as a cause of adult-acquired flatfoot deformity. Foot Ankle Int 2013;34:818–23.

24. Kann JN, Myerson MS. Intraoperative pathology of the posterior tibial tendon. Foot Ankle Clin 1997;2:343–54.

25. Chen JP, Allen AM. MR diagnosis of traumatic tear of the spring ligament in a pole vaulter. Skeletal Radiol 1997;26:310–2.

26. Weerts B, Warmerdam PE, Faber FWM. Isolated spring ligament rupture causing acute flatfoot deformity: case report. Foot Ankle Int 2012;33:148.

27. Borton DC, Saxby TS. Tear of the plantar calcaneonavicular (spring) ligament-causing flatfoot: a case report. J Bone Joint Surg Br 1997;79:641–3.

28. Houck JR, Neville CG, Tome J, et al. Ankle and foot kinematics associated with stage II PTTD during stance. Foot Ankle Int 2009;30(6):530–9.

29. Funk DA, Cass JR, Johnson KA. Acquired adult flat foot secondary to posterior tibial-tendon pathology. J Bone Joint Surg Am 1986;68(1):95–102.

30. Johnson KA, Strom DE. Tibialis posterior tendon dysfunction. Clin Orthop 1989; 239:196–206.

31. Jennings MM, Christensen JC. The effects of sectioning the spring ligament on rearfoot stability and posterior tibial tendon efficiency. J Foot Ankle Surg 2008; 47:219–24.

32. De la Portilla CC, Larrainzar-Garijo R, Bayod J. Biomechanical stress analysis of the main soft tissues associated with the development of adult acquired flatfoot deformity. Clin Biomech 2019;61(1):163–71.

33. MacDonald A, Cifo D, Knapp E, et al. Peritalar Kinematic changes associated with increased spring ligament tear in cadaveric flatfoot model. Foot Ankle Orthop 2018;3(3):1149–57.

34. Pasapula C, Devany A, Magan A, et al. Neutral heel lateral push test: the first clinical examination of spring ligament integrity. Foot (Edinb) 2015;25:69–74.

35. Pasapula C, Kiliyanpilakkil B, Khan DZ, et al. Plantar fasciitis: talonavicular instability/spring ligament failure as the driving force behind its histological pathogenesis. Foot 2021;101703.

36. Pasapula C, Al-Sukaini A, Band H, et al. Spring ligament insufficiency and hallux valgus as independent risk factors for first ray instability. Foot 2021;48: 101818.

37. Pasapula C, Cutts S. Modern theory of the development of adult acquired flat foot and an updated spring ligament classification system. Clin Res Foot Ankle 2017; 5(3):247.

38. Pasapula C, Shariff S, West J, et al. Adult acquired flat foot: a new biomechanical classification for the deformity based on two point failure of the medial column. Clin Res Foot Ankle 2018;6.

39. Kulig K, Reischl SF, Pomrantz AB, et al. Smith RW Nonsurgical management of posterior tibial tendon dysfunction with orthoses and resistive exercise: a randomized controlled trial. Phys Ther 2009;89:26–37.

40. Chao W, Wapner KL, Lee TH, et al. Non-operative management of posterior tibial tendon dysfunction. Foot Ankle Int 1996;17(12):736–41.

41. Kitaoka HB, Luo ZP, Kura H, et al. Effect of foot orthoses on 3-dimensional kinematics of flatfoot: a cadaveric study. Arch Phys Med Rehabil 2002;83: 876–9.

42. Hirano T, McCullough MBA, Kitaoka HB, et al. Effects of foot orthoses on the work of friction of the posterior tibial tendon. Clin Biomech 2009;24:776–80.

43. Augustin JF, Lin SS, Berberian WS, et al. Non-operative treatment of adult acquired flat foot with the Arizona brace. Foot Ankle Clin 2003;8(3):491–502.

44. Alvarez RG, Marini A, Schmitt C, et al. Stage I and II posterior tibial tendon dysfunction treated by a structured non-operative management protocol: an orthosis and exercise program. Foot Ankle Int 2006;27(1):2–8.

45. Lin JL, Balbas J, Richardson EG. Results of non-surgical treatment of stage II posterior tibial tendon dysfunction: a 7- to 10-year. FollowupFoot Ankle Int 2008;29(8):525–30.

46. Krause F, Bosshard A, Lehmann O, et al. Shell brace for stage II posterior tibial tendon insufficiency. Foot Ankle Int 2008;29(11):1095–100.

47. Nielsen MD, Dodson EE, Shadrick DL, et al. Non-operative Care for the treatment of adult-acquired flatfoot deformity. Jour Foot Ankle Surg 2011;50:311–4.

48. Balen PF, Helms CA. Association of posterior tibial tendon injury with spring ligament injury, sinus tarsi abnormality, and plantar fasciitis on MR imaging. AJR Am J Roentgenol 2001;176(5):1137–43.

49. Al-Mohrej OA, Al-Kenani NS. Acute ankle sprain: conservative or surgical approach? EFORT Open Rev 2016;1:34–44.

50. Richie DH. Biomechanics and orthotic treatment of the adult acquired flatfoot. Clin Podiatr Med Surg 2020;37:71–85.

51. Kulig K, Burnfield JM, Reischl S, et al. Effect of foot orthoses on tibialis posterior activation in persons with pes planus. Med Sci Sports Exerc 2005;37(1):24–9.

52. Richie DH. Biomechanics and clinical analysis of the adult acquired flatfoot. Clin Podiatr Med Surg 2007;24:617–44.

53. Tome J, Nawoczenski DA, Flemister A, et al. Comparison of foot kinematics between subjects with posterior tibialis tendon dysfunction and healthy controls. J Orthop Sports Phys Ther 2006;36:635–44.

54. Ringleb SI, Kavros SJ, Kotajarvi BR, et al. Changes in gait associated with acute stage II posterior tibial tendon dysfunction. Gait Posture 2007;25:555–64.

55. Steindler A. The supinatory compensatory torsion of the forefoot in pes valgus. J Bone Joint Surg Am 1929;11(2):272–6.

56. Johnson JE, Sangeorzan BJ, de Cesar Netto C, et al. Consensus on indications for medial cuneiform opening wedge (Cotton) osteotomy in the treatment of progressive collapsing foot deformity. Foot Ankle Int 2020;41(10):p1289–91.

57. Ellis SJ, Yu JC, Williams BR, et al. New radiographic parameters assessing forefoot abduction in the adult acquired flatfoot deformity. Foot Ankle Int 2009;30: 1168–76.

58. Lin YC, Mhuircheartaigh JN, Lamb J, et al. Imaging of adult flatfoot: correlation of radiographic Measurements with MRI. AJR 2015;204:354–9.

59. Younger AS, Sawatzky B, Dryden P. Radiographic assessment of adult flatfoot. Foot Ankle Int 2005;26(10):p820–5.

60. Mengiardi B, Zanetti M, Sch€ottle PB, et al. Spring ligament complex: MR imaging–anatomic correlation and findings in asymptomatic subjects. Radiology 2005;237:242–9.

61. Kitaoka HB, Crevoisier XM, Harbst K, et al. The effect of custom-made braces for the ankle and hindfoot on ankle and foot kinematics and ground reaction forces. Arch Phys Med Rehabil 2006;87:130–5.

62. Neville C, Flemister AS, Houck JR. Effects of the AirLift PTTD brace on foot kinematics in subjects with stage II posterior tibial tendon dysfunction. J Orthop Sports Phys Ther 2009;39:201–9.

63. Neville C, Houck J. Choosing among 3 ankle-foot orthoses for a patient with stage II posterior tibial tendon dysfunction. J Orthop Sports Phys Ther 2009;39:816–24.

64. Neville C, Lemley FR. Effect of ankle-foot orthotic devices on foot kinematics in Stage II posterior tibial tendon dysfunction. Foot Ankle Int 2012;33:406–14.

65. Pisani G. The coxa pedis. J Foot Ankle Surg 1994;1:67–74.

66. Carlson JM, Berglund G. An effective orthotic design for controlling the unstable subtalar joint. Orthotics and Prosthetics 1979;33(1):39–49.

67. Neville C, Bucklin M, Ordway N, et al. An ankle-foot orthosis with a lateral extension reduces forefoot abduction in subjects with stage ii posterior tibial tendon dysfunction. Orthop Sports Phys Ther 2016;46(1):26–33.

68. Lim WL, Liau LL, Ng MH, et al. Current progress in tendon and ligament tissue engineering. Tissue Eng Regen Med 2019;16(6):549–71.

Nonoperative Management of the Achilles Tendon Insertion

Jeffrey E. McAlister, DPM, FACFAS

KEYWORDS

- Nonoperative treatments • Insertional Achilles • Calcaneal enthesophyte
- Shockwave • Regenerative medicine • Platelet-rich plasma • Orthotics
- Physical therapy

KEY POINTS

- Insertional Achilles tendinopathy is thought of as a compression phenomenon with the posterosuperior calcaneus and the anterior aspect of the Achilles unlike midsubstance, which is more of a tension mechanism.
- Early treatment modalities to reduce pain are typically centered on immobilization for a short course followed by isometric exercises. Night splints or night braces have been shown to not be efficacious.
- To improve the blood flow, potentiate viable cells, and improve tenocyte formation, the author supports the utility of platelet-rich plasma, extracorporeal shockwave treatments, and other advanced modalities for this pathologic condition.

PATHOPHYSIOLOGIC INTRODUCTION

Clear definitions of Achilles pathology now exist and have been described by van Dijk and colleagues[1] based on anatomic location and histopathology to create a more uniform understanding of this disease process. We focus on insertional Achilles tendinopathy (IAT) defined as symptoms located at the insertion of the Achilles tendon onto the calcaneus, bone spurs, and calcifications in the tendon proper at the insertion site. Differential diagnoses may include retrocalcaneal bursitis or superficial calcaneal bursitis.

IAT has long been associated with several key mechanical contributing factors such as posterior muscle group tightness, pronation of the foot and calcaneus, large calcaneal enthesophytes, or spurs. Several investigators have discussed microtears within the tendon that failed to heal secondary to poor vascularity, which can lead to chronic pain. These tears are caused by excessive loading during aggressive exercise, uphill

Phoenix Foot and Ankle Institute, 7301 East 2nd Street, Suite 206, Scottsdale, AZ 85251, USA
E-mail address: Jeff.mcalister@gmail.com

Clin Podiatr Med Surg 39 (2022) 477–487
https://doi.org/10.1016/j.cpm.2022.02.008 **podiatric.theclinics.com**

training, repetitive overuse, and/or reduced flexibility. Histologic analyses show poor healing and a lack of inflammatory cell response, which incites pain.[2] As excessive load increases with individual foot types, normal tendon becomes stress shielded and reactive tendinopathy occurs with tendon disrepair and degenerative tendinopathy.[3] These therapies play roles in the understanding of IAT and non-IAT as we try to understand the true pathophysiology and correction of these degenerative processes. Current trends in the understanding of the disease process are somewhat static with the addition of plantaris compression phenomenon,[4,5] which is described later, but our challenge has focused on minimally invasive less debilitating recovery processes focused on rehabilitation (**Fig. 1**).

CLINICAL PRESENTATION AND WORKUP

Patients can present with symptoms that have been described in other articles in this review but focus on distal Achilles tendinitis. Patient-reported symptoms include pain with exertional activities, pain after a period of rest, swelling, and pain with closed counter shoes. Often patients complain of pain at end range of dorsiflexion, that is, walking uphill or heel drops, and pain with zero drop shoes or barefoot-style footwear. Midportion, or midsubstance, Achilles tendinopathy is typically located 2 to 7 cm from the insertion whereby IAT is focused at the superior calcaneal insertion or at the distal calcaneus posteriorly. Upon physical examination, as expected, tenderness to palpation along the posterior superior margin of the calcaneus, edema noted as well to the area which may present on the medial lateral insertional flares of the tendon, if a superficial bursitis is present there will be a softer bursal tissue typically at the directly posterior margin. Pain with end range of dorsiflexion active and passive of the affected limb and with weight-bearing exercises.

Imaging typically constitutes standard 4 weight-bearing views of the foot, including a calcaneal axial view, to assess for various pathologies including progressive collapsing foot deformity, cavovarus deformity, tarsal coalitions, and tibiotalar and hindfoot arthritis. Clinicians will typically rule in posterior calcaneal enthesophytes with these radiographs to determine the longevity and severity of the pathology and potential need for surgical management. Furthermore, as technology has improved and nonoperative treatments are becoming popular, point-of-care ultrasound is an oft first line of advanced imaging, which can be performed quickly and routinely

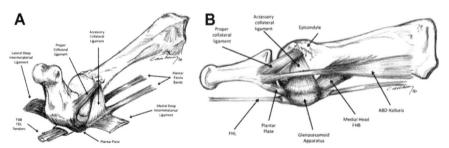

Fig. 1. Lateral weight-bearing foot radiograph with a focus on the posterior calcaneal enthesophyte, which is intratendinous at the Achilles insertion. *From* Caio Nery, Daniel Baumfeld, Hilary Umans, André F. Yamada, MR Imaging of the Plantar Plate: Normal Anatomy, Turf Toe, and Other Injuries, Magnetic Resonance Imaging Clinics of North America, Volume 25, Issue 1, 2017, Pages 127-144, ISSN 1064-9689, ISBN 9780323496537, https://doi.org/10.1016/j.mric.2016.08.007.

with a basic understanding of ultrasonic anatomy. If clinical symptoms continue despite nonoperative treatment or a better understanding of the patient's physiology is necessary, MRI is ordered and preferred. MRI typically allows for better visualization of the thickness of the tendon at the insertion as well as any outliers, which could include large amounts of bone marrow edema in the posterior superior calcaneal margin, stress fractures, bursal tissue, accessory soleus muscle, plantaris compression phenomenon, and posterior calcaneal fracture. These modalities will aid and guide treatment of IAT (**Fig. 2**).

PHASES OF TREATMENT
Pain Reduction

Because patients typically present after at least 6 to 8 weeks of at-home self-care, pain reduction is of utmost importance. These patients are on either side of the bell curve of activity, overuse phenomenon with runners or underuse and obese. Both are difficult to treat with their own challenges, but the former are often more difficult due to high expectations, need to return to sport activity, and lifestyle. The dysfunctional tendon at the insertion of the calcaneus is painful, and oral and topical anti-inflammatories combined with acetaminophen can assist. The author recommends acetaminophen 500 mg combined with 400 mg ibuprofen taken 3 times a day to begin treatment protocols and reduce tendon edema. Author recommends this course for approximately 4 weeks. This protocol also allows patient to begin isometric exercises, which is the functional exercise needed at this point in time. Isometric exercises help reduce pain and maintain Achilles tendon strength over this period. Simple calf raises on a flat surface repeated 3 to 5 times daily, which can be held for approximately 45 seconds, should be performed. Obviously aggravating cycles of Achilles tendon force should be removed, which include no running, jumping or box jumps, or impact activity for at least 3 to 4 weeks, but it may vary from patient to patient. The Achilles tendon is not to be stretched, passively, actively, or with bands or a night splint.

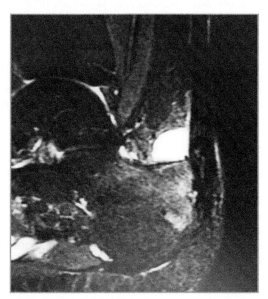

Fig. 2. Advanced imaging of posterior Achilles pain typically shows signal uptake anterior to the insertion and posterosuperior calcaneal edema on T2 MRI.

Oftentimes clinicians use a cam walker offloading boot to help with any difficulty with weight-bearing, but this also does not allow for functional recovery. The author recommends limiting the use of a Cam walker boot for 2 weeks before starting isometric exercises. After this phase of pain reduction modalities, approximately 4 weeks of the above-mentioned tools, the author recommends instituting advanced regenerative measures to include autologous injections (PRP, BMAC), nonautologous injections (HA), extracorporeal shockwave therapy (ESWT), percutaneous in-office procedures.

Intervention: Regenerative Therapies

At this phase in insertional Achilles tendinitis treatment, our goal is to change a chronic dysfunctional cytokine pathway and tendon disrepair to an acute inflammatory cell response that allows us to move forward with the next phase of building strength and return to sport.

AUTOLOGOUS INJECTIONS

Injections into the retrocalcaneal bursal tissue and around the calcaneal enthesophyte typically include platelet-rich plasma or bone marrow aspiration concentrate. The mechanism of action is increase in platelet activation at the site of injury, which causes growth factors, such as platelet-derived growth factor, to increase angiogenesis and macrophage activation at the site of injury. This increase in activation creates a process whereby the injection aids in local recruitment of macrophages and fibroblasts to repair damaged collagen, induction of angiogenesis, and blood vessel formation, as well as early inhibition of Cox-2.[6] Studies have waxed and waned over the last several years with a recent meta-analysis in 2018 revealing no significant difference in clinical outcome scores, tendon thickness, and color Doppler changes.[7] Erroi and colleagues[8] compared conservative treatment options commonly used: PRP and ESWT both combined with eccentric strengthening exercises. Visual analog scale (VAS) score and patient satisfaction improved in both studies over a 6-month follow-up. However, there was no statistically significant difference between the 2 combined treatments when compared with each other.[8] Iliac crest bone marrow aspirate injections have also been tabulated for treatment of recalcitrant cases. A recent study assessed 15 Achilles tendinopathies, 5 insertional, 8 noninsertional, and 2 combined, with an improvement over a 48-week follow-up. The investigators used a numeric rating system (NRS) pain score and recorded postoperative complications. No significant difference was seen between the various Achilles pathologies. Patients did demonstrate a statistically significant decrease in NRS pain score postoperatively.[9]

NONAUTOLOGOUS INJECTIONS

This category of injections would include high-volume injection (bupivacaine, normal saline, Depo-Medrol) and hyaluronic acid. A level 1 study assessing chronic Achilles tendinitis compared high-volume injection, PRP, and placebo in a randomized double-blinded prospective study. A total of 60 males were followed for 6 months with 3 arms of aforementioned treatment. Patients received 4 injections of the treatment as well as 12 weeks of daily eccentric strengthening program performed twice daily. The arm including the high-volume injection reported better patient outcomes in the short-term, although the 2 treatment arms plus eccentric strength training showed equivalent and best results at 6 months.[10] In a recent case series 29 patients with Achilles tendinitis received ultrasound-guided injections of hyaluronic acid, 40 mg/2.0 mL. Patient-reported outcomes were measured and recorded. Combined daily posterior chain strengthening exercises were recommended, and the patient followed a standard Alfredson protocol.[11] At 6-month follow-up personal satisfaction level was 69%, 48% of patients considered the result excellent, and AOFAS score improved from 71 to 90. There were no ruptures or complications. This study from Brazil adds to the body of knowledge that a nonautologous hyaluronic acid injection is a safe treatment option while improving function and reducing pain for 6 months. The exact mechanism of action is still being calculated in extra-articular roles; studies have shown a reduction in the inflammatory process and having a lubrication property.[12–16]

EXTRACORPOREAL SHOCKWAVE THERAPY

A concurrent treatment modality such as ESWT has been shown to be helpful in the treatment of IAT and non-IAT (**Fig. 3**). This regenerative option aims to enhance cell proliferation, migration, and secretory activity of tenocytes.[17] Also, ESWT can provide mechanical transduction, stimulating nitrous oxide and reducing pain and substance P and therefore inflammation. Studies to date have included too many variables or have been low level. A recent study examined the effectiveness of ESWT in the treatment of chronic IAT in a double-blind randomized sham controlled trial[18] the 2 groups being low-energy ESWT and sham arm. Radial shockwave of 2000 pulses was applied at the affected injury site once a week for 4 weeks with concurrent eccentric exercises. The patients were followed for 6 months. ESWT maintained significant improvements

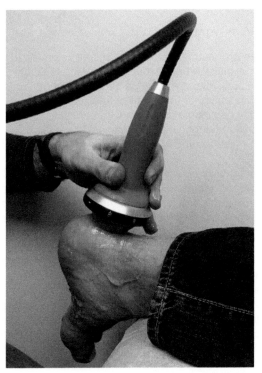

Fig. 3. Extracorporeal shockwave therapy performed in conjunction with isometric exercises has been shown to be clinically efficacious.

in VAS at weeks 4 through 12. This study maintained no significant difference in VAS scores at 6 months. Another study compared ESWT in active versus nonactive patients with a 5-year follow-up. This level 3 study retrospectively compared 33 patients by self-reported activity. At 5-year follow-up, the active patient population had significantly lower mean VAS scores (0.3 vs 1.6) and significantly higher mean patient-reported outcome scores compared with the control group. Of note there was no significant difference between the 2 groups regarding the ultrasonographic assessment of the insertion sites.[19] The investigators found that "sports activity level is an important factor influencing long-term ESWT outcomes for IAT." A large, level 1, randomized controlled trial from Brazil assessed the challenges of differentiating variables. This study aimed to assess again, whether ESWT aids in the outcome of IAT treatment with eccentric exercises. A total of 119 patients were included and placed into 2 different treatment arms. The first treatment arm included eccentric exercises with ESWT, and the second treatment arm was a control group with a sham shockwave therapy unit. Patient-reported outcomes were followed over a period of 24 weeks. Both groups improved in patient-reported outcomes, although there was no between-group difference in any of the outcomes. The investigators found that ESWT did not potentiate the effects of eccentric strengthening in chronic IAT.[20]

A recent systematic review of nonoperative treatment modalities assessed 23 studies over the past 17 years. The investigators found that a combination treatment such as ESWT and eccentric exercises has a grade B recommendation versus isolated treatments. Superiority of 1 combination over another could not be confirmed, although support of the eccentric exercises in combination with more studies needed to confirm autologous injection therapy or other soft tissue treatments.[21]

MINIMALLY INVASIVE TREATMENTS

This section focuses on treatment modalities before returning to sport and activity, which include minimal incision treatments and evolving technologies that attempt to improve tendon function. These typically go hand in hand with regenerative medicine techniques during this phase of treatment before returning to sport. Again, IAT has taught us to treat this pathologic condition with a multiheaded approach and insert eccentric strengthening throughout the progress.

Two such technologies include radiofrequency coblation and ultrasonic percutaneous tenotomy.

The goal of radiofrequency coblation (aka microdebrider) is to induce degeneration of sensory nerve fibers, introduce long-term angiogenic responses, ablate pain without sacrificing the structure or strength of the tendon, and have an antinociceptive effect.[22,23] This treatment has been shown to improve VAS scores and a oh FAS score is at 6 months in chronic foot and ankle tendinosis including Achilles, peroneal and posterior tibial tendinitis[24] radiofrequency procedures may shorten the natural history of the disease process and hasten recovery. Radiofrequency coblation is typically performed in the office under local anesthesia or even in the operating room under moderate sedation. The author recommends using a prone technique, which allows full visualization of the proposed site. Preoperatively marking out the site of pain assists with topographic anatomy. The author also recommends using regenerative injections such as platelet-rich plasma or bone marrow aspirate concentrate during this procedure to assist with biologic improvements (**Fig. 4**). Multiple small incisions are made with an 18-gauge needle down to the level of the Achilles tendon through peritenon. The radiofrequency coblation wand is then inserted through each incision, and the tip is placed intrasubstance. A study of 47 cases with a mean follow-up of 8.6 months

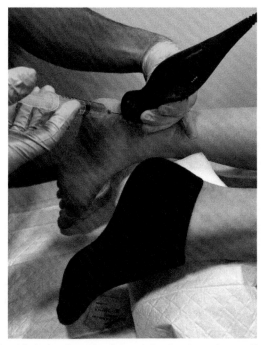

Fig. 4. Ultrasound-guided platelet-rich plasma injection into the medial Achilles insertion and retrocalcaneal bursa.

showed a 15% reoperation rate and 12% rate of Achilles rupture. The investigators found that a high body mass index should raise caution for immediate weight-bearing and possibly delayed this protocol.[25] Most studies have focused on midsubstance Achilles tendinosis, and with higher rates of complications some surgeons have avoided aggressive radiofrequency coblation treatments. There are no specific head-to-head studies assessing open debridement versus radiofrequency coblation and eccentric exercises. This procedure or combination of procedures may possibly be best for high-risk patients with wound healing complications. Further studies are warranted to prove its effectiveness and efficacy.

Ultrasonic percutaneous tenotomy is typically performed as stated under ultrasound guidance. This technology depends on a cavitation principle whereby the goal is to remove or excise damaged or diseased tissue, which creates bubbles because of diseased cell lysis, and this is debrided with continuous suction irrigation. Very few studies exist in the literature, and most are case series or case reports. Some animal bench studies show improvements in collagenase after histologic analysis.[26] Similar to radiofrequency coblation, this process can be performed in a procedure room or under local anesthesia in the office. Patients are typically weight-bearing as tolerated in a cam walker boot for approximately 2 weeks while the tendon heals. After this, eccentric exercises are instituted in a controlled fashion with physiotherapy. Two studies recently highlighted a retrospective review of patient's home had ultrasonic percutaneous tenotomy's. The studies highlighted that a high learning curve is present and that with little experience clinicians can remove too much healthy tendon or fail to remove all of the pathologic tendon. There is also an increased risk of poor healing potential and vascularity. The investigators highlighted a 70% satisfaction rate with no ruptures documented. This study had a nearly 2-year follow-up postprocedure.[27,28] A recent systematic review of percutaneous ultrasonic tenotomies revealed very little evidence in the long term and only modest improvement in the short term[29] (**Fig. 5**).

Again, these treatments for IAT are typically used in conjunction, and more evidence is needed to fully support more invasive procedures. Phase 1 includes pain reduction with anti-inflammatories and oftentimes controlled isometric exercises. Phase 2 or intervention phase includes regenerative options to stimulate a chronic process and promote macrophage activity while promoting angiogenesis. If minimally invasive treatments are performed a period of immobilization is typically supported for 2–4 weeks depending on the case. As the team progresses into building strength and returning to sport, it is important to use physical therapy as a tool for guidance and progression.

Return to Sport/Activity

Progression into sport needs to be slow and progressive. The aforementioned treatments aimed to increase the vascularity and improve tendon function, and at this point strengthening needs to ensue. Eccentric insertional Achilles exercises are continued with avoidance of dorsiflexion loading. Patients are encouraged to perform 3 sets of 15 to 20 reps twice per day, 7 d/wk, 12 weeks with progression. Heavy load is progressed as symptoms resolve. Focusing on soleus and gastrocnemius strength work is important. Mild symptoms may occur during exercise, and as long as they are settling the day after, patients can resume exercise. The goal is to return to sport

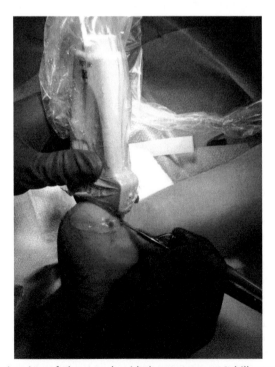

Fig. 5. Intraoperative view of ultrasound-guided percutaneous Achilles tenotomy, which attempts to remove damaged and diseased tendon from healthy tenocytes. More studies are needed to show efficacy.

after 6 weeks of treatment, but a gradual return is recommended especially to high-impact activities such as running. Obviously at this point appropriate shoe gear is implemented to have a larger heel counter and avoidance of "0 drop" or flat shoe gear. Various studies have proved the ineffectiveness of night splints, taping, and foot orthoses in the treatment of IAT.[30,31]

Nonoperative treatment of insertional Achilles tendinitis is challenging and poses daily struggles in many foot and ankle specialists' offices. This tendinopathy is commonplace in the active and nonactive patient demographics. Specifically Taylor treatments are important and have been proved to include pain reduction, intervention of choice, and a slow progression to return to activity. More evidence is needed to support minimally invasive or percutaneous options described earlier. As with any foot and ankle tendinopathy or pathology, failure to concede to nonoperative treatment typically starts at around 6 months depending on the duration. At that point in time patients are typically ready for advanced, operative techniques. These will later be elucidated in detail.

CLINICS CARE POINTS

- Understand the nomenclature associated with Achilles tendinitis
- No more "Haglund deformity"
- Nonoperative treatment typically needs to fail over a course of 3 to 6 months before prior to surgical intervention
- Three phases of treatment: pain reduction, regenerative/reparative therapies, return to sport/activity
- Follow Alfredon protocol for Achilles tendinopathy
- Return to sport slowly and gradually, letting pain rest below a 5

DISCLOSURE

The author has nothing to disclose.

REFERENCES

1. van Dijk CN, van Sterkenburg MN, Wiegerinck JI, et al. Terminology for Achilles tendon related disorders. Knee Surg Sports Traumatol Arthrosc 2011;19(5): 835–41.
2. Kujala UM, Sarna S, Kaprio J. Cumulative incidence of achilles tendon rupture and tendinopathy in male former elite athletes. Clin J Sport Med 2005;15(3): 133–5.
3. September AV, Cook J, Handley CJ, et al. Variants within the COL5A1 gene are associated with Achilles tendinopathy in two populations. Br J Sports Med 2009;43(5):357–65.
4. Masci L, Neal BS, Wynter Bee W, et al. Achilles Scraping and plantaris tendon removal improves pain and tendon structure in patients with mid-Portion achilles tendinopathy-A 24 Month follow-up case series. J Clin Med 2021;10(12):2695.
5. Alfredson H, Masci L, Spang C. Ultrasound and surgical inspection of plantaris tendon involvement in chronic painful insertional Achilles tendinopathy: a case series. BMJ Open Sport Exerc Med 2021;7(1):e000979. https://doi.org/10.1136/bmjsem-2020-000979.

6. Monto RR. Platelet rich plasma treatment for chronic Achilles tendinosis. Foot Ankle Int 2012;33(5):379–85.

7. Zhang YJ, Xu SZ, Gu PC, et al. Is platelet-rich plasma injection effective for chronic achilles tendinopathy? A meta-analysis. Clin Orthop Relat Res 2018; 476(8):1633–41.

8. Erroi D, Sigona M, Suarez T, et al. Conservative treatment for Insertional Achilles Tendinopathy: platelet-rich plasma and focused shock waves. A retrospective study. Muscles Ligaments Tendons J 2017;7(1):98–106.

9. Thueakthong W, de Cesar Netto C, Garnjanagoonchorn A, et al. Outcomes of iliac crest bone marrow aspirate injection for the treatment of recalcitrant Achilles tendinopathy. Int Orthop 2021;45(9):2423–8.

10. Boesen AP, Hansen R, Boesen MI, et al. Effect of high-volume injection, platelet-rich plasma, and sham treatment in chronic Midportion achilles tendinopathy: a randomized double-blinded prospective study. Am J Sports Med 2017;45(9): 2034–43.

11. Alfredson H, Pietilä T, Jonsson P, et al. Heavy-load eccentric calf muscle training for the treatment of chronic Achilles tendinosis. Am J Sports Med 1998;26(3): 360–6.

12. Kumai T, Muneta T, Tsuchiya A, et al. The short-term effect after a single injection of high-molecular-weight hyaluronic acid in patients with enthesopathies (lateral epicondylitis, patellar tendinopathy, insertional Achilles tendinopathy, and plantar fasciitis): a preliminary study. J Orthop Sci 2014;19(4):603–11.

13. Ayyaswamy B, Vaghela M, Alderton E, et al. Early outcome of a single Peri-Tendinous hyaluronic acid injection for mid-Portion Non-insertional achilles tendinopathy - a pilot study. Foot (Edinb) 2021;49:101738.

14. Petrella RJ, Cogliano A, Decaria J. Combining two hyaluronic acids in osteoarthritis of the knee: a randomized, double-blind, placebo-controlled trial. Clin Rheumatol 2008;27(8):975–81.

15. Lee GW, Seo HY, Jung DM, et al. Comparison of Preoperative bone Density in patients with and without Periprosthetic Osteolysis following Total ankle Arthroplasty. Foot Ankle Int 2021;42(5):575–81.

16. Ferreira GF, Caruccio FRC, Guerrero Bou Assi JR, et al. Ultrasound-guided hyaluronic acid injection for the treatment of insertional Achilles tendinopathy: a prospective case series. Foot Ankle Surg 2021. https://doi.org/10.1016/j.fas.2021. 12.004. S1268-7731(21)00244-7.

17. Visco V, Vulpiani MC, Torrisi MR, et al. Experimental studies on the biological effects of extracorporeal shock wave therapy on tendon models. A review of the literature. Muscles Ligaments Tendons J 2014;4(3):357–61.

18. Pinitkwamdee S, Laohajaroensombat S, Orapin J, et al. Effectiveness of extracorporeal shockwave therapy in the treatment of chronic insertional achilles tendinopathy. Foot Ankle Int 2020;41(4):403–10.

19. Zhang S, Li H, Yao W, et al. Therapeutic response of extracorporeal shock wave therapy for insertional achilles tendinopathy between sports-active and Nonsports-active patients with 5-year follow-up. Orthop J Sports Med 2020; 8(1). 2325967119898118.

20. Mansur NSB, Matsunaga FT, Carrazzone OL, et al. Shockwave therapy plus eccentric exercises versus isolated eccentric exercises for achilles insertional tendinopathy: a double-blinded randomized clinical trial. J Bone Joint Surg Am 2021;103(14):1295–302.

21. Zhi X, Liu X, Han J, et al. Nonoperative treatment of insertional Achilles tendinopathy: a systematic review. J Orthop Surg Res 2021;16(1):233.

22. Takahashi N, Tasto JP, Ritter M, et al. Pain relief through an antinociceptive effect after radiofrequency application. Am J Sports Med 2007;35(5):805–10.
23. Ochiai N, Tasto JP, Ohtori S, et al. Nerve regeneration after radiofrequency application. Am J Sports Med 2007;35(11):1940–4.
24. Yeap EJ, Chong KW, Yeo W, et al. Radiofrequency coblation for chronic foot and ankle tendinosis. J Orthop Surg (Hong Kong) 2009;17(3):325–30.
25. Shibuya N, Thorud JC, Humphers JM, et al. Is percutaneous radiofrequency coblation for treatment of Achilles tendinosis safe and effective? J Foot Ankle Surg 2012;51(6):767–71.
26. Kamineni S, Butterfield T, Sinai A. Percutaneous ultrasonic debridement of tendinopathy-a pilot Achilles rabbit model. J Orthop Surg Res 2015;10:70. https://doi.org/10.1186/s13018-015-0207-7.
27. Sanchez PJ, Grady JF, Saxena A. Percutaneous ultrasonic tenotomy for achilles tendinopathy is a surgical procedure with Similar complications. J Foot Ankle Surg 2017;56(5):982–4.
28. Chimenti RL, Stover DW, Fick BS, et al. Percutaneous ultrasonic tenotomy reduces insertional achilles tendinopathy pain with high patient satisfaction and a low complication rate. J Ultrasound Med 2019;38(6):1629–35.
29. Vajapey S, Ghenbot S, Baria MR, et al. Utility of percutaneous ultrasonic tenotomy for Tendinopathies: a systematic review. Sports Health 2021;13(3):258–64.
30. Scott LA, Munteanu SE, Menz HB. Effectiveness of orthotic devices in the treatment of Achilles tendinopathy: a systematic review. Sports Med 2015;45(1):95–110.
31. Wilson F, Walshe M, O'Dwyer T, et al. Exercise, orthoses and splinting for treating Achilles tendinopathy: a systematic review with meta-analysis. Br J Sports Med 2018;52(24):1564–74.

Operative Management
Plantar Plate

Brett D. Sachs, DPM, FACFAS[a,b,]*, Laura B. Adler, DPM[b],
Robert J. Cavaliere, DPM[b]

KEYWORDS

- Crossover toe • Lesser metatarsophalangeal joint instability • Metatarsalgia
- Plantar plate • Predislocation syndrome

KEY POINTS

- The main goals of operative management of plantar plate pathologies are to restore function, reduce deforming forces, and regain static and dynamic stability about the lesser metatarsophalangeal joint (MPJ).
- Plantar plate pathology can be addressed using a variety of different surgical techniques. These include direct, indirect, dorsal, plantar, and arthroscopic approaches.
- In addition to local deforming forces about the MPJ, one should consider rearfoot driven and suprapedal deformities when performing a comprehensive surgical evaluation and work-up.

INTRODUCTION

The plantar plate is a vital structure for maintaining lesser metatarsophalangeal joint (MPJ) stability.[1] Its primary role is to provide static stabilization of the MPJs, working in conjunction with the long and short flexor and extensor tendons. When insufficiency or attenuation of the plantar plate occurs, a sagittal plane deformity will slowly develop, eventually leading to a "crossover toe" transverse plane deformity.[2]

Coughlin coined this descriptive term to describe the later stages of deformity, most commonly affecting the second MPJ.[2] Shortly after, Yu and Judge elaborated on this condition describing it as "predislocation syndrome"; an inflammatory condition affecting the plantar plate causing pain and instability, which could progress to subluxation at the MPJ.[3]

BACKGROUND

Histologic analysis of the plantar plate tissue has outlined not only its anatomic characteristics, but has helped with our understanding of its role in regards to function. The

[a] Rocky Mountain Foot & Ankle Center, 7615 W. 38th Avenue, Suite B101, Wheat Ridge, CO 80033, USA; [b] Highlands-Presbyterian, St. Luke's Podiatric Medicine and Surgery Residency Program, 1719 East 19th Avenue, Denver, CO 80218, USA
* Corresponding author.
E-mail address: bdsachs@hotmail.com

Clin Podiatr Med Surg 39 (2022) 489–502
https://doi.org/10.1016/j.cpm.2022.02.009
0891-8422/22/© 2022 Elsevier Inc. All rights reserved.

podiatric.theclinics.com

plantar plate is composed of mainly fibrocartilaginous tissue, with contributions from the plantar aponeurosis as well as the MPJ joint capsule.

It is composed of both type I and type II collagen, contributing to its structural integrity and fibrocartilaginous nature. The presence of this type I collagen and fibrocartilaginous tissue is what allows the plantar plate to endure the repetitive stresses that are placed on it.

The plantar plate has multiple attachments to the MPJ complex, firmly adhered to the proximal phalangeal base and loosely adhered to the associated metatarsal neck. It also serves as an attachment point for the deep transverse metatarsal ligaments as well as the plantar fascia and intrinsic musculature (**Fig. 1**). These contributions allow for this structure to maintain congruence between the metatarsal head and phalangeal base because there are no direct long or short flexor attachments in this area. Its size is variable and depends on its anatomic location, measuring approximately 20 mm in length, 16 mm in width, and 2 to 5 mm in thickness.[4] The plantar plate acts as the principal static stabilizer of the MPJ, integral to the overall stability of the proximal phalanx and digit.

Injury to the plantar plate frequently occurs secondary to trauma, inflammatory arthritides, or chronic synovitis.[4] This is commonly related to altered forefoot, hindfoot, or suprapedal pathomechanic forces. Pathology can occur along any part of the plantar plate and can be seen with both acute and chronic causes. Hallux valgus and digital contractures are often seen in association with plantar plate injuries.[5] Hammertoe deformities cause retrograde forces that place increased pressure on the metatarsal and soft tissue structures. An elongated second metatarsal, or shortened first metatarsal, have also been proposed as a predisposing factor for attenuation of the plantar plate[6] (**Fig. 2**).

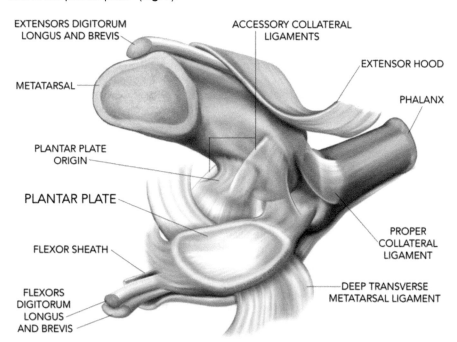

Fig. 1. Anatomy of the plantar plate. (*From* Chris Mallac, Plantar plate tear: a common overload injury in athletes, Ankle and foot injuries, Diagnose & Treat, https://www.sportsinjurybulletin.com/plantar-plate-tear-a-common-overload-injuryin-athletes/)

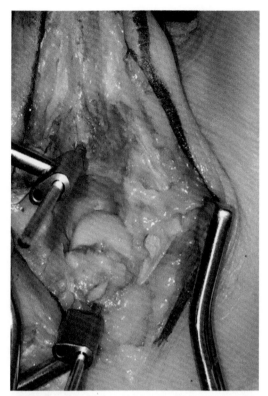

Fig. 2. Chronic attenuation of the plantar plate. Notice the degenerative tissue in the central portion of the plantar plate.

Thompson and Hamilton stated that a relatively short first metatarsal combined with an elongated second metatarsal causes overload of the second MPJ.[7] Similarly, equinus and first ray hypermobility or insufficiency seen in hallux abducto valgus deformity may lead to forefoot overload resulting in plantar plate attenuation or rupture (**Fig. 3**). Other associated predisposing pathologic conditions include hallux limitus/rigidus, medial column instability, and disruption of the plantar joint capsule. Common presentations include the gradual onset of pain and swelling of the plantar MPJ with loss of toe purchase.[5]

PREVALENCE

The population most commonly affected by plantar plate pathology consists of sedentary women aged 50 to 70 years and athletic men aged 25 to 60 years. The former, is thought to be secondary to high-heeled shoe gear, whereas the latter is likely affected secondary to weakening of periarticular structures due to repetitive trauma.[3,8] Although typically seen in the second ray, Nery and colleagues[9] reported findings on 55 plantar plate tears in which two-thirds of patients had second toe involvement and one-third of patients had third toe involvement.

PATIENT EVALUATION OVERVIEW

Patients with plantar plate patholgy typically present with plantar pain about the affected MPJ that subsides with rest, swelling of the MPJ, and the sensation of

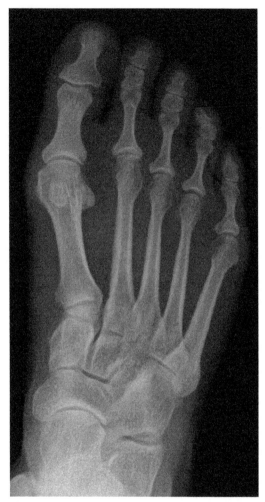

Fig. 3. Radiograph demonstrating long second metatarsal with hallux abducto valgus deformity.

walking on a bruise or lump. Patients may also report the feeling of dislocation or malposition of the toe with ambulation. The pain and swelling is most commonly located distal to the affected metatarsal head and MPJ area.[8] This location correlates with the most common location of plantar plate tears where it inserts onto the proximal phalanx base. This was described by Blitz and colleagues[10] as the "rupture zone." Symptoms may vary based on severity and timing with acute presentations being less common. Klein and colleagues[11] reported that 93% of patients reported insidious onset of pain in comparison to 7% with acute onset of pain. Although not every patient with plantar plate patholgy will present with deformity, earlier cases may sometimes present with subtle dislocation of the MPJ or early lack of toe purchase. More chronic cases tend to progress toward complete subluxation and MPJ dislocation. Over time, as the plantar plate and collateral ligaments further attenuate, the affected digit may deviate in the sagittal and coronal planes and crossover or even under the neighboring digit. A crossover toe deformity was found to have a high specificity for plantar plate tears or attenuation.[7,11]

PHYSICAL EXAMINATION

Several clinical tests have been described in diagnosing plantar plate tears. Thompson and Hamilton described the "vertical stress test," "drawer test," or "Lachman test," which is positive if there is more than 2-mm of dorsal displacement of the phalanx on a stabilized metatarsal or greater than 50% of MPJ subluxation. This test is considered pathognomonic for plantar plate pathology and MPJ instability.[8] Pain and inflammation at the second MPJ along with a positive drawer test identified 95% of patients with plantar plate pathology correlated with intraoperative findings.[11]

Nery and colleagues[12] also presented a classification system based on the degree of MPJ subluxation ranging from grade 0 to the most severe, grade 4, being a complete dislocation at the MPJ. Bouche and Heit described the "paper pull-out test" where the patient is asked to stand and resist a strip of paper being pulled from beneath the toe by plantarflexing the affected digit. A failure to resist the paper being pulled is considered a positive test.[8,9] Both of these tests correlate with the clinical examination finding seen as loss of toe purchase on weight-bearing examination. Another common but nonspecific finding is edema localized at the MPJ as well as pain on palpation to the base of the proximal phalanx or plantar to the affected metatarsal head. As stated previously, conditions that predispose patients to increased forefoot pressures place the plantar plate at risk. It is important to evaluate concomitant pathologic conditions in order to address all contributing factors in order to optimize patient outcomes. Evaluation of the first ray and assessment of hypermobility or rigidity is imperative in order to understand the pathophysiology causing plantar plate injury and prevent recurrence. Ankle range of motion and a Silfverskiold test should also be performed to evaluate for equinus, which may need to be addressed as well. Patients' symptoms are often nonspecific and may be attributed to other conditions. For this reason, advanced imaging, such as an ultrasound or magnetic resonance imaging (MRI) can help further delineate the involvement of the plantar plate versus other causes of pain and discomfort. Differential diagnoses include intermetatarsal neuroma, metatarsalgia, synovitis, arthritis, insufficiency fracture, avascular necrosis, fat pad atrophy, and chondral injuries.[13]

IMAGING

Standard foot radiographs should be included in every patient workup. Radiographs will allow the surgeon to evaluate the overall foot structure as well as the metatarsal parabola. Typical findings for plantar plate pathology include dorsal joint dislocation or transverse plane deviation of the affected toe (**Fig. 4**). It has been shown that medial deviation is more common than lateral deviation.[13]

Radiographs can also be used for other pathologic conditions such as arthritic changes, first ray pathology, stress fracture, and Freiberg infarction. Contralateral views may be helpful for comparison in less obvious cases. Imaging combined with a complete history and physical is usually sufficient in diagnosing a plantar plate injury. Some more difficult cases may benefit from advanced imaging methods, including MRI, ultrasound or arthrography.

An MRI study can be useful to detect plantar plate tears (**Fig. 5**). In 2 studies assessing plantar plate tears, experienced musculoskeletal radiologists evaluated MRIs and found a specificity of 100%. In 2 recent studies, MRIs have been shown to have a sensitivity of 74% to 95%.[13–15] In a study by Yamada and colleagues, the authors

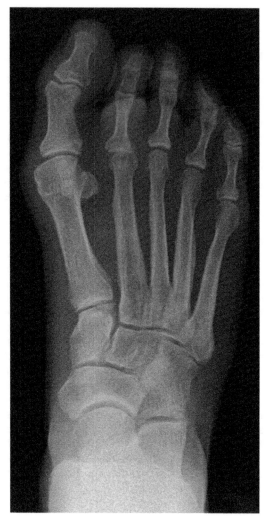

Fig. 4. Radiograph demonstrating a dislocated second toe secondary to an acute plantar plate tear.

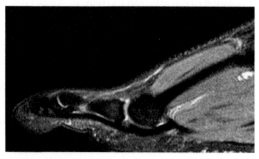

Fig. 5. Plantar plate tear on MRI T2-weighted image as indicated by the red arrow.

correlated MRI features with intraoperative findings of plantar plate tears. The presence of pericapsular fibrosis had a sensitivity of 91.2% and specificity of 90.9%.[16] Although MRI is very useful, an ultrasound may be more cost effective. Although both modalities are dependent on technique, each imaging study can play a role in diagnosing difficult plantar plate injuries.

Plantar plate defects on ultrasound will be seen as loss of homogeneity and replacement of normal echoic tissue with hypoechoic tissue.[15] In a study comparing MRI and ultrasound with intraoperative findings of plantar plate defects, the authors found that the sensitivity, specificity, positive predictive value and negative value of MRI were 73.9%, 100%, 100%, and 29.4% compared with ultrasound, which was 91.5%, 25%, 91.5%, and 25%, respectively.[15] They found that an MRI was more helpful in localizing plantar plate pathology in grade II and III tears, whereas ultrasound was better able to detect these tears.[15]

Another modality, which is less commonly used, is arthrography. This technique requires injection of a radiopaque contrast dye into the affected MPJ to evaluate for contrast extension. Contrast in the flexor sheath is diagnostic of a plantar plate rupture.[13]

OPERATIVE MANAGEMENT

There are a myriad of treatment options for plantar plate pathology and injuries. Conservative treatment options commonly include a trial of splinting, padding, activity modification, physical therapy, nonsteroidal anti-inflammatory drugs (NSAIDs), corticosteroid injections, and orthotics. Surgical intervention may be warranted if conservative measures are unsuccessful. Surgical treatment options include direct or indirect repair of the plantar plate and can be performed by a dorsal approach, plantar approach, or a combination of each (**Fig. 6**). Arthroscopy of the MPJ and radiofrequency shrinkage have also been described.[17] The 2 most common procedures used to indirectly address plantar plate repair (PPR) is the metatarsal shortening

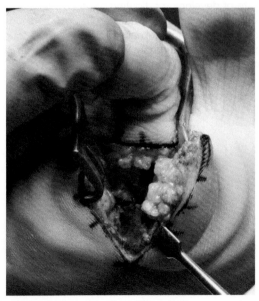

Fig. 6. Direct repair of the plantar plate through a plantar approach.

osteotomy of the affected metatarsal (**Fig. 7**) and the Girdlestone–Taylor flexor to extensor tendon transfer[5,10] (**Fig. 8**). These procedures can be performed alone or in combination and work to indirectly address the deformity by decompressing the joint and plantarflexing the digit. A metatarsal shortening osteotomy also allows for better visualization and access to the plantar plate when performing a direct repair. In 2015, Sung described a technique of reconstructing the plantar plate using a synthetic suture tape and interference screws in the metatarsal head and proximal phalanx.[18] The suture is tensioned until digital purchase is achieved to recreate MPJ stability. This technique can be helpful in patients with attenuated tissue or complete ruptures of the plantar plate. It allows for repair of the direct plantar plate while sparing the flexor tendons.[18] Another procedure that has been described to repair a second digit crossover toe deformity combines a minimally invasive technique of plantar plate tenodesis with extensor digitorum brevis (EDB) tendon transfer.[19] The tenodesis corrects the sagittal plane deformity, whereas the EDB transfer corrects the transverse plane deformity. The authors also used a 1.9 mm 30° arthroscope to assess the plantar plate and confirm integrity of its proximal phalanx attachment. The use of arthroscopy has the added benefit of joint evaluation and assessing for possible intra-articular pathology.

Another less commonly performed surgical option that indirectly addresses the plantar plate is a lesser MPJ arthrodesis. However, there are only a few published reports evaluating outcomes of lesser MPJ arthrodesis for PPR.

COMPLICATIONS

In general, surgical management to address plantar plate attenuation is relatively successful, offering favorable outcomes and pain relief. There are, however, many reports of commonly encountered complications. These include floating toe, joint stiffness, overcorrection or undercorrection of the toe, nerve or vascular compromise, recurrence of the deformity, arthritis of the MPJ, and transfer metatarsalgia. The most prevalent complication associated with this type of procedure is the floating toe deformity. The complication rate of developing a floating toe following a shortening metatarsal osteotomy has been reported in the literature up to 36% and with a recurrence rate of 15%.[20] In a study by Migues and colleagues,[21] the authors found that the floating toe deformity was seen more commonly when performed with concomitant digital procedures such as the proximal interphalangeal joint arthrodesis. The flexor tendon

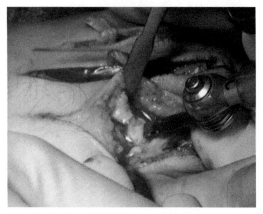

Fig. 7. Performing a second metatarsal shortening osteotomy.

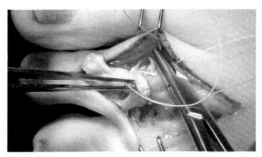

Fig. 8. Flexor digitorum longus tendon transfer. The figure shows suturing of the flexor tendon to the extensor digitorum longus tendon.

transfer has been shown to result in postoperative stiffness, and patient satisfaction following this procedure ranges in the literature from 51% to 89%.[10] The frequency in complications of these mainstay procedures led to the development in direct PPR techniques. Several techniques for plantar incisional approaches to PPR have been described in the literature including a linear intermetatarsal space incision and "L"-shaped incision. The concern for hypertrophic or painful scars of the plantar foot as well as wound healing issues may be a factor in choosing a dorsal versus a plantar approach.[5] Sharpe and colleagues, retrospectively, assessed the rate of complications in 204 direct plantar approach PPRs. They reported an overall complication rate of 15%. The complications included a superficial infection rate of 6.8%, painful plantar scars in 8.3%, and 1.4% reoperation rate.[22]

NEW DEVELOPMENTS

Although there has not been any significant recent advancement on plantar plate reconstruction technology to our knowledge, there are several systems on the market to repair the plantar plate. Most recently, an anchor implant composed of suture has been released which has the advantage of being performed through dorsal or plantar approaches and can be fixated into soft tissue or bone (Paratrooper, Paragon28, Denver, CO). Another relatively new soft tissue fixation system (TenoTac, Paragon28, Denver, CO) has emerged, which can be used in place of a flexor to extensor tendon transfer. This device uses a 2-piece cannulated, titanium implant, which allows the surgeon to fixate the flexor tendons against the proximal phalanx to achieve sagittal and/or transverse plane stability. Benefits of this technique include the ability to dial in correction using either the long and/or short flexor tendons. Another more recent repair system for direct PPR is the Gravity system (Wright Medical, Memphis, TN). This system includes corkscrew needle passers attached to nonabsorbable suture, which makes it easier to pass suture through this small area. Finally, the HAT-TRICK lesser toe repair system (Smith + Nephew, Memphis, TN) and the Complete Plantar Plate Repair (CPR; Arthrex, Naples, FL) use a specialized suture passer to perform a direct primary repair of the plantar plate through a dorsal approach.

EVALUATION OF OUTCOME AND/OR LONG-TERM RECOMMENDATIONS

In a study by Flint and colleagues,[23] the authors performed a Weil osteotomy with PPR through a dorsal approach and assessed functional and patient reported outcomes. The authors used the CPR System (Arthrex, Naples, FL) or Viper system (Arthrex, Naples, FL) to repair the plantar plate. They evaluated 97 feet with 138 PPRs, with only 15 of those being isolated PPRs. Although there was no significant difference, the patients with isolated PPRs showed 100% satisfaction, self-rated as good to excellent. The patients with Weil osteotomy and PPR reported good to excellent results in 80.4% (78/97), fair in 15.5% (15/97), and poor in 4.1% (4/97).[23]

The mean american orthopedic foot and ankle score (AOFAS) increased significantly from 49 points preoperatively to 81 points at 12-month follow-up. The isolated PPR subgroup showed an increase in AOFAS from 46 to 85.[23] It is well established that a long second metatarsal has been found to be an etiologic risk factor for plantar plate pathology and metatarsalgia. Fleischer and colleagues[24] compared a direct plantar plate approach combined with a Weil osteotomy to a Weil osteotomy alone for these patients. They evaluated patients 1 year postoperatively and found that patients in the Weil osteotomy and PPR group had higher quality of life and improved pain FAOS scores compared with the Weil osteotomy group alone. Second digit alignment was similar between groups in both sagittal and transverse plane radiographs. The authors graded patient's plantar plate tears using Nery classification, and found that the Weil/PPR group had higher grade tears (median grade 3) compared with the isolated Weil group (median grade 1). The Weil/PPR group also had a significantly higher body mass index (BMI) in comparison with the Weil group. The authors concluded that combining PPR with a Weil osteotomy may be helpful regardless of the grade of plantar plate tear.[24]

In separate studies performed by Bouché and Prissel, the authors performed direct PPR via a plantar approach and found that 27% to 33% of patients lacked toe purchase at final follow-up.[5,23] Bouche combined his PPR with an FDL transfer, which resulted in increased stiffness, whereas Prissel used a shortening metatarsal osteotomy in nearly 60% of patients through a separate plantar incision.[5,25] In a retrospective, case controlled study by Cook and colleagues,[26] the authors compared direct PPR through a dorsal approach with soft tissue rebalancing procedures. Their soft tissue component included various combinations, which consisted of flexor tendon transfer, capsulotomy, capsulorrhaphy, tendon and skin lengthening procedures among several others. They concluded that anatomic PPR resulted in 94% digital stability compared with 60% in the soft tissue-rebalancing group.[26] In a meta-analysis evaluating the flexor tendon transfer procedure, the authors found the procedure to have an overall patient satisfaction rate of 91.8% when including prospective articles of high quality.[27] They found increased rates of satisfaction when performed in conjunction with a PIPJ arthrodesis. The main complaint following flexor tendon transfer was stiffness of the operative toe.[27] In a cadaver study by Ford and colleagues[28], the authors compared a direct PPR with a flexor tendon transfer. They concluded that the combination of direct PPR with tendon transfer was optimal for MPJ stabilization.[28] A cadaveric study by Chalayon assessed the biomechanics of PPR via a Weil shortening osteotomy, a flexor tendon transfer, or a combination of the 2 and conclude that the combination of the metatarsal osteotomy with a flexor tendon transfer best restored the stability of the MPJ against subluxation and dorsiflexory forces.[29]

In a small case series evaluating 4 patients with 5 extensively dislocated lesser MPJs, the authors performed a lesser MPJ arthrodesis procedure. The patients had various causes leading to significant deformity. The authors positioned the MPJ at 0° in the frontal and transverse plane and 5 to 15° in the sagittal plane to align with the adjacent digits using a dorsal locking plate.[30] There were several other adjunctive procedures performed concurrently, including hallux interphalangeal joint arthrodesis, first MPJ arthrodesis, hammertoe correction, and soft tissue procedures. There were 2 patients who required local wound care; one for superficial necrosis of the digit and the other for a wound dehiscence. There was one nonunion that went on to revision

Table 1	
Anatomic grading system for plantar plate injury	
Injury Grade	**Anatomic Findings**
0	Plantar plate or capsular attenuation with or without dislocation
I	Transverse distal tear adjacent to insertion into proximal phalanx (<50%); medial, central, or lateral area with or without midsubstance tear
II	Transverse distal tear (>50%); medial, central, or lateral area with or without midsubstance tear
III	Transverse and/or longitudinal extensive tear; may involve collateral ligaments
IV	Extensive tear with button hole (dislocation); transverse and longitudinal plate tear combined

and successful fusion. All patients achieved union clinically and radiographically at a mean time of 16.4 weeks and patients had a mean follow-up of 21 months.[30] In a study by Karlock, 11 patients underwent second MPJ arthrodesis using a k-wire and staple construct. At 19-month follow-up, 10 patients had good to excellent results and one patient had a poor result. Ten of the patients went on to successful union with one asymptomatic nonunion, one minor wound dehiscence which resolved, and one distal proximal phalanx shaft fracture.[31] The author concluded that this procedure may be useful for those with severe, rigid deformities and low activity demands.[31] Although the arthrodesis procedure can be successful in treating severely dislocated MPJs, these are small studies with short-term follow-up. Currently, there are no long-term studies or controlled trials and further research is needed to recommend this procedure.

Nery and colleagues, evaluated patients prospectively and created a protocol for surgical treatment based on the grading of the plantar plate tear. The authors graded the pathology intraoperatively and performed radiofrequency ablation with thermal shrinkage for grade 0–I, direct repair on the plantar plate in grade II–III, and a Girdlestone–Taylor procedure for grade IV (**Table 1**). They also performed concomitant Weil osteotomies in all cases. There was a significant improvement in all groups in terms of clinical and radiographic parameters. They found patients with grade 0 and II plantar plate pathology had superior results with more stable MPJs compared with grades I, II, and IV.[32] The authors performed arthroscopy using a 2.7 mm 30° scope to grade the plantar plates and also performed synovectomies when needed.

SUMMARY

The plantar plate is a vital structure contributing to the stability of the lesser MPJs. Its fibrocartilaginous nature, abundant in type I collagen, is essential to its ability to withstand the robust forces that are placed on it. Early recognition of an injury to the plantar plate allows the clinician to trial conservative modalities. In later presentations of plantar plate pathology , surgical intervention might be warranted. When evaluating the integrity of the plantar plate, one must recognize not only local deforming forces but suprapedal forces as well. For superior outcomes, surgical planning must localize and address these deforming forces. Newer technology and advancement of established techniques allow the surgeon to not only decrease the morbidity associated with surgical intervention but decrease the risk of recurrence, as well.

CLINICS CARE POINTS

- Its important to do a thorough work-up to confirm a plantar plate tear or rupture and develop an appropriate treatment plan
- A positive drawer test is highly specific for a plantar plate abnormality
- In order to ensure long-term success, one must address all deforming forces and associated deformities to stabilize the second MPJ and prevent overload

---

DISCLOSURE

[1] The authors have nothing to disclose as it relates to the content of this article.

REFERENCES

1. Blazek CD, Brandão RA, Manway JM, et al. Multiplanar correction of the lesser digital deviation and indirect plantar plate rupture repair using a braided polyethylene Nylon suture: a technique guide. Foot Ankle Spec 2017;10(6):551–4.
2. Coughlin MJ. Crossover second toe deformity. Foot Ankle 1987;8(1):29–39.
3. Yu GV, Judge MS, Hudson JR, et al. Predislocation syndrome: progressive subluxation/dislocation of the lesser metatarsophalangeal joint. J Am Podiatr Med Assoc 2002;92(4):182–99.
4. Watson TS, Reid DY, Frerichs TL. Dorsal approach for plantar plate repair with Weil osteotomy: operative technique: operative technique. Foot Ankle Int 2014; 35(7):730–9.
5. Prissel MA, Hyer CF, Donovan JK, et al. Plantar plate repair using a direct plantar approach: an outcomes analysis. J Foot Ankle Surg 2017;56(3):434–9.
6. Mann TS, Nery C, Baumfeld D, et al. Is second metatarsal protrusion related to metatarsophalangeal plantar plate rupture? AJR Am J Roentgenol 2021;216(1): 132–40.
7. Thompson FM, Hamilton WG. Problems of the second metatarsophalangeal joint. Orthopedics 1987;10(1):83–9.
8. Doty JF, Coughlin MJ. Metatarsophalangeal joint instability of the lesser toes. J Foot Ankle Surg 2014;53(4):440–5.
9. Nery C, Coughlin MJ, Baumfeld D, et al. Lesser metatarsophalangeal joint instability: prospective evaluation and repair of plantar plate and capsular insufficiency. Foot Ankle Int 2012;33(4):301–11.
10. Blitz NM, Ford LA, Christensen JC. Plantar plate repair of the second metatarsophalangeal joint: technique and tips. J Foot Ankle Surg 2004;43(4):266–70.
11. Klein EE, Weil L Jr, Weil LS Sr, et al. Clinical examination of plantar plate abnormality: a diagnostic perspective: a diagnostic perspective. Foot Ankle Int 2013; 34(6):800–4.
12. Nery C, Coughlin M, Baumfeld D, et al. How to classify plantar plate injuries: parameters from history and physical examination. Rev Bras Ortop 2015;50(6): 720–8.
13. Hsu RY, Barg A, Nickisch F. Lesser metatarsophalangeal joint instability: advancements in plantar plate reconstruction. Foot Ankle Clin 2018;23(1):127–43.

---

[1] Confirm Dr. Sachs' disclosures

14. Sung W, Weil L Jr, Weil LS Sr, et al. Diagnosis of plantar plate injury by magnetic resonance imaging with reference to intraoperative findings. J Foot Ankle Surg 2012;51(5):570–4.

15. Klein EE, Weil L Jr, Weil LS Sr, et al. Magnetic resonance imaging versus musculoskeletal ultrasound for identification and localization of plantar plate tears. Foot Ankle Spec 2012;5(6):359–65.

16. Yamada AF, Crema MD, Nery C, et al. Second and third metatarsophalangeal plantar plate tears: diagnostic performance of direct and indirect MRI features using surgical findings as the reference standard. AJR Am J Roentgenol 2017; 209(2):W100–8.

17. Nery C, Raduan FC, Catena F, et al. Plantar plate radiofrequency and Weil osteotomy for subtle metatarsophalangeal joint instability. J Orthop Surg Res 2015 Nov 19;10:180.

18. Sung W. Technique using interference fixation repair for plantar plate ligament disruption of lesser metatarsophalangeal joints. J Foot Ankle Surg 2015;54(3): 508–12.

19. Lui TH. Correction of crossover deformity of second toe by combined plantar plate tenodesis and extensor digitorum brevis transfer: a minimally invasive approach. Arch Orthop Trauma Surg 2011;131(9):1247–52.

20. Highlander P, VonHerbulis E, Gonzalez A, et al. Complications of the Weil osteotomy. Foot Ankle Spec 2011;4(3):165–70.

21. Migues A, Slullitel G, Bilbao F, et al. Floating-toe deformity as a complication of the Weil osteotomy. Foot Ankle Int 2004;25(9):609–13.

22. Sharpe BD Jr, Ebaugh MP, Prissel MA, et al. Direct plantar approach to plantar plate repair and associated wound complications. Foot Ankle Orthop 2020; 5(4). 2473011420S0043.

23. Flint WW, Macias DM, Jastifer JR, et al. Plantar plate repair for lesser metatarsophalangeal joint instability. Foot Ankle Int 2017;38(3):234–42.

24. Fleischer AE, Klein EE, Bowen M, et al. Comparison of combination Weil metatarsal osteotomy and direct plantar plate repair versus Weil metatarsal osteotomy alone for forefoot metatarsalgia. J Foot Ankle Surg 2020;59(2):303–6.

25. Bouché RT, Heit EJ. Combined plantar plate and hammertoe repair with flexor digitorum longus tendon transfer for chronic, severe sagittal plane instability of the lesser metatarsophalangeal joints: preliminary observations. J Foot Ankle Surg 2008;47(2):125–37.

26. Cook JJ, Johnson LJ, Cook EA. Anatomic reconstruction versus traditional rebalancing in lesser metatarsophalangeal joint reconstruction. J Foot Ankle Surg 2018;57(3):509–13.

27. Iglesias ME, Vallejo RB, Jules KT. Meta-analysis of flexor tendon transfer for the correction of lesser toe deformities. J Am Podiatr Med Assoc 2012 Sep-Oct; 102(5):359–68.

28. Ford LA, Collins KB, Christensen JC. Stabilization of the subluxed second metatarsophalangeal joint: flexor tendon transfer versus primary repair of the plantar plate. J Foot Ankle Surg 1998;37(3):217–22.

29. Chalayon O, Chertman C, Guss AD, et al. Role of plantar plate and surgical reconstruction techniques on static stability of lesser metatarsophalangeal joints: a biomechanical study: a biomechanical study. Foot Ankle Int 2013;34(10): 1436–42.

30. Hollawell SM, Kane BJ, Paternina JP, et al. Lesser metatarsophalangeal joint pathology addressed with arthrodesis: a case series. J Foot Ankle Surg 2019;58(2): 387–91.

31. Karlock LG. Second metatarsophalangeal joint fusion: a new technique for cross-over hammertoe deformity. A preliminary report. J Foot Ankle Surg 2003;42(4): 178–82.
32. Nery C, Coughlin MJ, Baumfeld D, et al. Prospective evaluation of protocol for surgical treatment of lesser MTP joint plantar plate tears. Foot Ankle Int 2014; 35(9):876–85.

Operative Management
Spring Ligament

Jacob Jones, DPM[a], Alan Catanzariti, DPM, FACFAS[b],*

KEYWORDS

- Spring ligament • Adult acquired flatfoot • Posterior tibial dysfunction

KEY POINTS

- The spring ligament is the most important static stabilizer of the medial column.
- Spring ligament disease is directly associated with posterior tibial tendon disease.
- Reconstruction of the spring ligament is a reasonable ancillary procedure that supports anatomic reduction of peritalar subluxation.
- Reconstruction of the spring ligament augmented with suture tape provides increased stability and maintenance of correction under cyclical loading.
- Reconstruction of the spring ligament should be protected with extra-articular osteotomies to correct the deforming forces that resulted in the tear.

INTRODUCTION

Pes planovalgus is a multiplanar deformity consisting of a combination of hindfoot valgus, collapse of the medial longitudinal arch, forefoot varus, and forefoot abduction. This deformity is often associated with posterior tibial tendon dysfunction.[1] Collapse of the medial longitudinal arch increases stress to the static stabilizers of the medial column including the deltoid ligament, spring ligament, plantar fascia, plantar and talocalcaneal interosseous ligaments, as well as the talonavicular and naviculocuneiform capsules.[2] There is a higher incidence of concomitant spring ligament pathologic condition in pes planovalgus deformity and posterior tibial tendon dysfunction based on magnetic resonance imaging and intraoperative observation, compared with other static stabilizers.[3]

The spring ligament is composed of a superomedial calcaneonavicular and inferior calcaneonavicular components.[4] The superomedial component includes the medial

[a] Resident Physician, Department of Orthopedics, Division of Foot & Ankle Surgery, West Penn Hospital, Foot & Ankle Institute, 4800 Friendship Avenue N1, Pittsburgh, PA 15224, USA; [b] West Penn Hospital Foot & Ankle Surgery, Section Chief of Podiatry, Department of Orthopedic Surgery, Allegheny Health Network, 4800 Friendship Avenue N1, Pittsburgh, PA 15224, USA
* Corresponding author. Foot & Ankle Institute, West Penn Hospital, 4800 Friendship Avenue N1, Pittsburgh, PA 15224.
E-mail address: alan.catanzariti@ahn.org

Clin Podiatr Med Surg 39 (2022) 503–519
https://doi.org/10.1016/j.cpm.2022.02.010
0891-8422/22/© 2022 Elsevier Inc. All rights reserved.

talonavicular capsule and is composed of both fibrous and fibrocartilaginous tissues. This portion of the spring ligament is the largest and strongest portion of the complex and is an important static stabilizer of the talonavicular joint, which resists development of pes planovalgus deformity.[3,4]

Spring ligament reconstruction is used as an adjunctive procedure in adult acquired flatfoot reconstruction, and various techniques have been described. These techniques include the use of the posterior tibial tendon, flexor halluces longus tendon, peroneus longus tendon, and direct repair with augmentation.[5–10] Biomechanical studies have demonstrated that suture tape augmentation of spring ligament reconstruction strengthens the repair with cyclical loading in cadaveric specimens.[11] Spring ligament reconstruction can be a powerful adjunctive procedure that obviates the need nonanatomic techniques or arthrodesis, as it allows for anatomic reduction of peritalar subluxation.[5]

PATIENT EVALUATION

Adult acquired flatfoot deformity can be classified using the description originally described by Johnson and Strom and later modified by Myerson.[12,13] The Myerson classification system can be found in **Table 1**.

It is difficult to discern spring ligament disruption based on clinical examination alone and evaluation of the spring ligament through advanced imaging can be useful.[3,14] Deland and colleagues described the following grading system for MRI evaluation of ligamentous structures in adult acquired flatfoot: grade 0, an intact ligament with uniform hypointense signal intensity; grade I, degeneration, denoted with MRI as increased signal intensity involving less than 50% of the cross-sectional area of the ligament on axial images; grade II, degeneration of more than 50%; grade III, a partial tear with less than 50% of the fibers discernible on MRI with both increased signal intensity and abnormal morphology; and grade IV, a tear involving abnormal morphology of more than 50% of the cross-sectional area.[3] In this study, Deland and colleagues found that the spring ligament was the most commonly affected ligament in posterior tibial tendon dysfunction. They also noted that the degree of spring ligament disease was equivalent to that of posterior tibial tendon disease.[3]

SURGICAL APPROACH

The patient is positioned in a supine position with a bump under the ipsilateral hip. Extra-articular osteotomies should be performed as necessary in order to remove the deforming forces and offload the medial longitudinal arch. Following realignment osteotomies, the surgeon may proceed with repairing the static and dynamic stabilizers of the medial longitudinal arch.

A standard medial longitudinal incision for posterior tibial tendon repair and flexor digitorum longus transfer is made from the tip of the medial malleolus to the medial cuneiform (**Fig. 1**). The posterior tibial tendon sheath is identified and incised to expose the tendon (**Fig. 2**). The posterior tibial tendon is evaluated and explored. Although the integrity of the posterior tibial tendon must be thoroughly investigated, the most important aspect of posterior tibial tendon preservation is excursion of the tendon (**Fig. 3**). If there is adequate excursion of the posterior tibial tendon, the diseased portions of the tendon may be excised and the tendon repaired. However, if excursion is inadequate, the posterior tibial tendon should be excised. The spring ligament may be evaluated by retracting the posterior tibial tendon to expose the superomedial component of the spring ligament complex.

Table 1
Myerson flatfoot deformity classification[17]

Stage	Clinical Manifestation	Clinical Findings	Radiographic Manifestations	Conservative Treatment	Surgical Treatment
Stage I	Tenosynovitis of the PTT or partial rupture without deformity	Intact single heel rise, intact inversion resistance with foot in plantarflexion	Normal alignment or mild hindfoot valgus	Immobilization, NSAIDs	Tenosynovectomy, calcaneal osteotomy, midfoot stabilization, or osteotomy
Stage IA	Inflammatory disease causes PTT rupture (ie, rheumatoid arthritis)	Hindfoot alignment maintained	Normal alignment	Immobilization, NSAIDs	Tenosynovectomy
Stage IB	Partial PTT rupture with normal hindfoot alignment	Hindfoot alignment maintained	Normal alignment	NSAIDs, immobilization	Tenosynovectomy with or without calcaneal osteotomy
Stage IC	Partial PTT rupture with hindfoot valgus	Slight hindfoot valgus deformity (5° or less)	Slight hindfoot valgus	NSAIDs, immobilization	Tenosynovectomy, medial translational calcaneal osteotomy, medial column stabilization or osteotomy
Stage II	PTT rupture or tendinosis	Clinically apparent flatfoot deformity, inability to perform a single heel raise, weakness with inversion	Hindfoot valgus, loss of calcaneal pitch, forefoot abduction, forefoot supination, medial column instability	Orthoses, NSAIDs, physical therapy	Extra-articular osteotomies, posterior tibial tendon repair, FDL tendon transfer, spring ligament repair, subtalar joint arthrodesis, peroneus brevis to longus tendon transfer
Stage IIA	Flexible hindfoot valgus with minimal forefoot supination	Reducible hindfoot valgus deformity	Hindfoot valgus without forefoot abduction	Orthoses, NSAIDs, physical therapy	FDL tendon transfer, PTT repair or allograft, medializing calcaneal osteotomy, subtalar joint arthrodesis, peroneus brevis to longus tendon transfer, medial column arthrodesis, or osteotomy

(continued on next page)

Table 1
(continued)

Stage	Clinical Manifestation	Clinical Findings	Radiographic Manifestations	Conservative Treatment	Surgical Treatment
Stage IIB	Flexible hindfoot valgus with flexible forefoot supination	Forefoot supination reduces with foot in plantarflexion and hindfoot valgus reduced	Hindfoot valgus without forefoot abduction	Orthoses, NSAIDs, physical therapy	Gastrocnemius recession, FDL tendon transfer, PTT repair or allograft, medializing calcaneal osteotomy, subtalar joint arthrodesis, peroneus brevis to longus tendon transfer, medial column arthrodesis, or osteotomy
Stage IIC	Flexible hindfoot valgus with fixed forefoot supination	Forefoot remains supinated with foot in plantarflexion and hindfoot reduced to neutral	Hindfoot valgus without forefoot abduction	Orthoses, NSAIDs, physical therapy	Gastrocnemius recession, FDL tendon transfer, PTT repair or allograft, medializing calcaneal osteotomy, subtalar joint arthrodesis, peroneus brevis to longus tendon transfer, medial column arthrodesis, or osteotomy
Stage IID	Flexible hindfoot valgus with forefoot abduction	Hindfoot valgus with abduction resulting in too many toes sign	Hindfoot valgus with forefoot abduction due to TMT arthritis or secondary to hindfoot deformity	Orthoses, NSAIDs, physical therapy	Primary deformity is the TMT: TMT arthrodesis with FDL tendon transfer Primary deformity is hindfoot: TMT arthrodesis with lateral column lengthening and FDL tendon transfer

Stage				Orthoses, NSAIDs, physical therapy	
Stage IIE	Flexible hindfoot valgus with medial column instability	Dorsiflexion of the medial column with hindfoot valgus, subtalar joint impingement	Hindfoot valgus without forefoot abduction	Orthoses, NSAIDs, physical therapy	Lateral column lengthening, medial cuneiform osteotomy, spring ligament reconstruction, TMT arthrodesis, NC arthrodesis, TN arthrodesis when >50% TN uncoverage
Stage III	PTT rupture with rigid hindfoot valgus with or without rigid forefoot abduction	Inability to perform single heel rise, significant weakness with inversion, medial longitudinal arch does not reconstitute	Loss of subtalar joint space, loss of talonavicular joint space, hindfoot valgus, forefoot abduction	Custom bracing	Double arthrodesis, triple arthrodesis, lateral column lengthening
Stage IIIA	Rigid hindfoot valgus without forefoot abduction	Rigid hindfoot valgus	Hindfoot valgus with loss of subtalar joint space, loss of talonavicular joint space, hindfoot abduction	Custom bracing	Double or triple arthrodesis
Stage IIIB	Rigid hindfoot valgus with forefoot abduction	Rigid hindfoot valgus with forefoot abduction	Hindfoot valgus with loss of subtalar joint space, loss of talonavicular joint space, hindfoot and forefoot abduction	Custom bracing	Double arthrodesis with lateral column lengthening or triple arthrodesis with bone block CCJ arthrodesis
Stage IV	Ankle valgus	Ankle valgus with flexible or rigid hindfoot valgus, possible medial ankle instability	Ankle valgus	Custom bracing	Deltoid reconstruction, calcaneal osteotomies, midfoot and hindfoot arthrodesis, gastrocnemius recession, tibiotalocalcaneal arthrodesis, pantalar arthrodesis, ankle arthrodesis

(continued on next page)

Table 1
(continued)

Stage	Clinical Manifestation	Clinical Findings	Radiographic Manifestations	Conservative Treatment	Surgical Treatment
Stage IVA	Flexible ankle valgus	Reducible ankle valgus with or without associated hindfoot deformity	Ankle valgus	Custom bracing	Deltoid reconstruction, calcaneal osteotomies, midfoot/hindfoot arthrodesis
Stage IVB	Rigid ankle valgus	Irreducible ankle valgus	Ankle valgus	Custom bracing	Ankle arthrodesis, pantalar arthrodesis, tibiotalocalcaneal arthrodesis, hindfoot arthrodesis with medial ankle reconstruction staged with total ankle arthroplasty

PTT, posterior tibial tendon; NSAIDs, non-steroidal anti-inflammatory; FDL, flexor digitorum longus; MRI, magnetic resonance imaging.
Data from Myerson MS, Kadakia AR. Reconstructive foot and ankle surgery management. Philadelphia, PA: Elsevier Saunders. 2005.

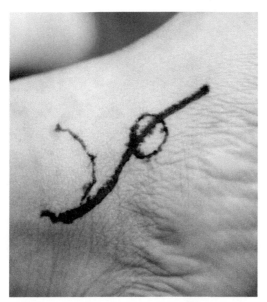

Fig. 1. Curvelinear incision from the tip of the medial malleolus to the medial cuneiform.

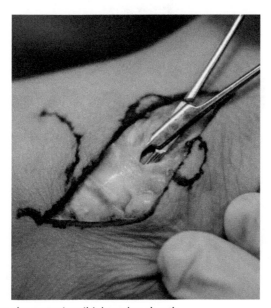

Fig. 2. Incision into the posterior tibial tendon sheath.

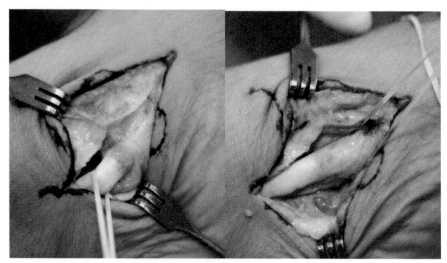

Fig. 3. Identification and inspection of the posterior tibial tendon.

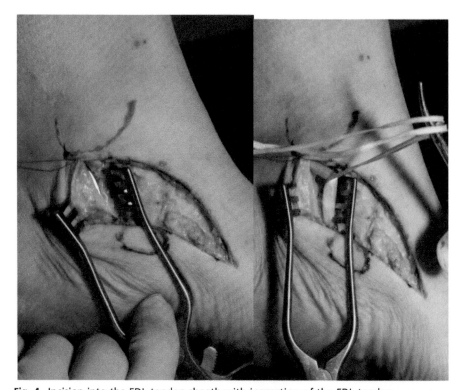

Fig. 4. Incision into the FDL tendon sheath with inspection of the FDL tendon.

PRIMARY REPAIR OF SPRING LIGAMENT

Primary repair of the spring ligament may be performed when adequate soft tissue is present and the ends of the ligament can be reapproximated. This should be completed with the foot in a neutral position and with care taken to avoid knot irritation against the posterior tibial tendon.

SURGICAL RECONSTRUCTION WITH FLEXOR DIGITORUM LONGUS TENDON TRANSFER AND AUGMENTATION

The flexor digitorum longus tendon sheath is identified and incised (**Fig. 4**). The FDL is transected distally near the knot of Henry to allow for adequate tendon length for transfer. The FDL tendon is then whipstitched in standard fashion to allow for tenodesis (**Fig. 5**).

The superomedial aspect of the spring ligament complex should be evaluated. Any tears or attenuation of the ligament should be directly repaired. Repair of the diseased ligament should be augmented in order to provide necessary stability of the medial longitudinal arch. The authors commonly use a dual arm suture tape for augmentation of their repair. This is completed by inserting an anchor into the

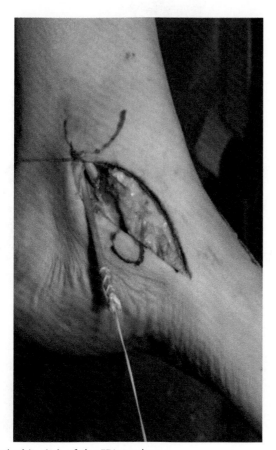

Fig. 5. Harvest and whipstitch of the FDL tendon.

sustentaculum tali with care taken to avoid the subtalar joint (**Figs. 6** and **7**). A drill-hole is then created from plantar to dorsal through the navicular tuberosity with care taken to maintain the medial bone bridge. The size of the drillhole should be determined by the size of the FDL tendon because this drillhole will also be used for the tendon transfer.

One arm of the suture tape is passed from dorsal to plantar through the drillhole (**Fig. 8**). The second arm of the suture tape is passed from plantar to dorsal through the drillhole. The FDL is also passed through the drillhole from plantar to dorsal (**Fig. 9**). The plantar arm of the suture tape should be tensioned as much as possible. The dorsal arm of the suture tape should be tensioned until the talonavicular joint is reduced. The suture tape arms and FDL tendon are secured in place with a single tenodesis screw inserted into the plantar aspect of the navicular drillhole (**Figs. 10** and **11**).

A cadaveric study by Aynardi and colleagues found that this fixation construct with augmentation was superior to direct repair in cyclical loading. In their study, cyclical loading resulted in a 100% failure rate in the direct repair cohort compared with a

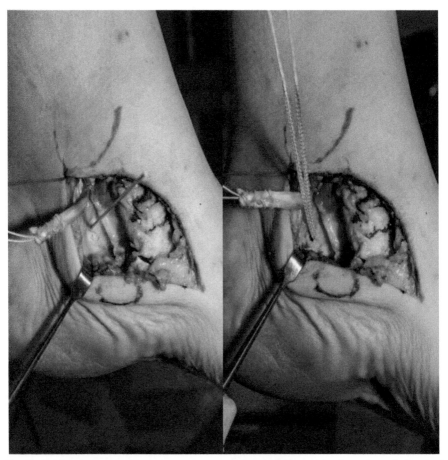

Fig. 6. Guide pin inserted into the sustentaculum tali followed by insertion of the dual armed suture tape.

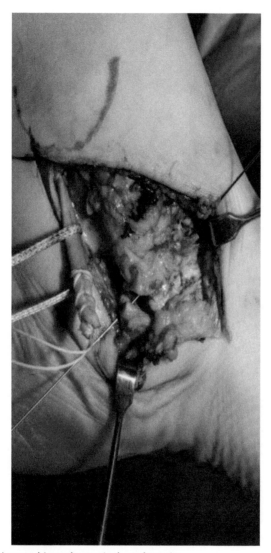

Fig. 7. Guide pin inserted into the navicular tuberosity.

13% failure rate in the augmentation cohort. Additionally, they found a greater maintenance of Meary angle at peak forces in the augmentation cohort.[11]

SURGICAL RECONSTRUCTION WITH PERONEUS LONGUS AUTOGRAFT

Spring ligament reconstruction with peroneus longus tendon transfer has been described.[15] In order to use the peroneus longus, the surgeon must ensure that the peroneus longus and peroneus brevis tendons are in relatively free of pathologic condition, and that bony realignment does not result in overcorrection. The peroneus longus tendon is harvested through a lateral incision along the fibula. The surgeon must

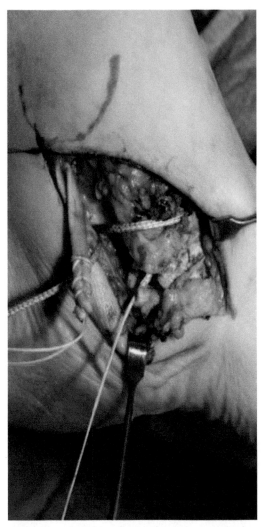

Fig. 8. Suture arm passed from dorsal to plantar through navicular bone tunnel.

ensure that adequate tendon is harvested to complete the reconstruction. The proximal aspect of the peroneus longus tendon is transferred to the peroneus brevis.

A navicular bone tunnel is placed from dorsal to plantar, whereas a tibial bone tunnel is placed from the inferior midportion of the medial malleolus and exits medially approximately 5 cm proximal to the ankle joint. A separate incision is made along the medial tibia to allow for appropriate tensioning of the graft.

The peroneus longus tendon is passed from dorsal to plantar through the navicular bone tunnel along the medial aspect of the talar head and through the tibia bone tunnel. It is tensioned with the foot held in neutral position with slight adduction. The tendon is first secured to the navicular and then appropriately tensioned before securing to the tibia. Fixation can be achieved with tenodesis screws or through whip-stitch secured to a screw on the dorsal navicular and proximal tibia bone tunnel exit.

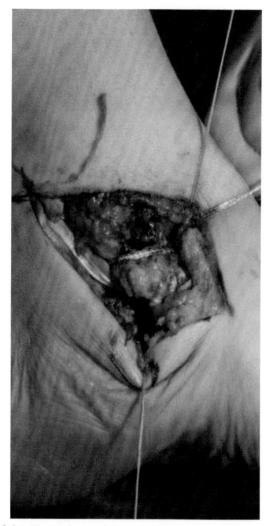

Fig. 9. Insertion of the FDL tendon and second suture arm from plantar to dorsal through navicular bone tunnel.

This fixation construct also allows for reconstruction of the superficial deltoid, which is not uncommonly involved in adult acquired flatfoot.[15].

POSTOPERATIVE CARE

Patients are to remain nonweight bearing in a posterior splint or short leg cast for 6 weeks. Patients may then transition to protected weight bearing in a walking boot for 2 to 3 weeks. Patients then gradually transition to standard footwear and undergo a short course of functional rehabilitation. This post-operative protocol may be altered depending on concomitant procedures performed.

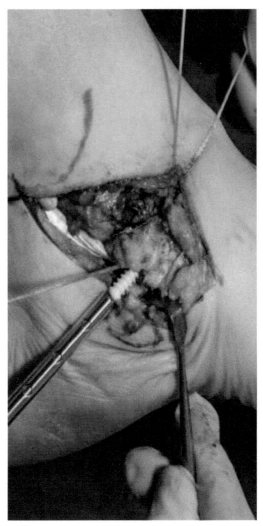

Fig. 10. Insertion of a biotenodesis screw from plantar to dorsal to secure tendon transfer and suture arms.

OUTCOMES

Spring ligament reconstruction is commonly performed as an adjunctive procedure in posterior tibial tendon dysfunction and adult acquired flatfoot deformity. Therefore, it is difficult to ascertain the outcomes of the reconstruction techniques. In a recent study by Xu and colleagues, they analyzed anatomic and nonanatomic spring ligament reconstruction techniques in isolation. They found that nonanatomic reconstruction techniques provided the greatest correction of hindfoot and midfoot alignments in adult acquired flatfoot deformity.[16] The literature describing differing reconstruction techniques emphasize the importance of boney realignment in order to protect the soft tissue reconstruction. An isolated reconstruction of the spring ligament complex will not adequately realign the hindfoot or midfoot deformities.[5–11,15]

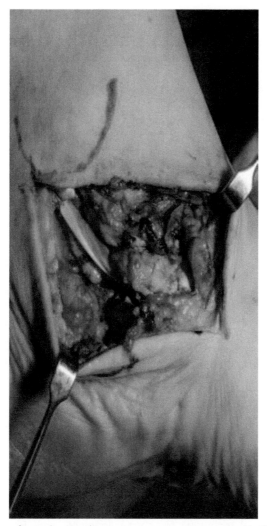

Fig. 11. Tendon transfer and spring ligament reconstruction augmentation secured.

SUMMARY

Spring ligament reconstruction is a powerful adjunctive procedure in the treatment of posterior tibial tendon dysfunction and adult acquired flatfoot deformity. The spring ligament is an important static stabilizer of the medial longitudinal arch, especially resisting deformity at the talonavicular joint.[3,4] Isolated spring ligament reconstruction will not correct deformities of the hindfoot and midfoot. Such deformities much be corrected with osseous realignment procedures, which will also protect the spring ligament repair.[5–11,15] When performing spring ligament reconstruction, it is important to augment the repair in order to improve the stability of the reconstruction.[11] Finally, nonanatomic reconstruction techniques may provide greater stability and correction when compared with anatomic repairs.[16]

CLINICS CARE POINTS

- Spring ligament disruption should be evaluated in patients with posterior tibial tendon disease.
- Spring ligament disease evaluation can be done through MRI or intraoperative inspection.
- Surgical repair of the spring ligament is a valuable adjunctive procedure in posterior tibial tendon dysfunction and flatfoot reconstruction, however, it should be performed in addition to deformity correction with osseous realignment procedures.

DISCLOSURE

The authors have nothing to disclose.

REFERENCES

1. Funk DA, JRh Cass, Johnson KA. Acquired adult flat foot secondary to posterior tibial tendon pathology. J Bone Joint Surg Am 1986;68:95–102.
2. Raikin SM, Winters BS, Daniel JN. The RAM classification. Foot Ankle Clin N Am 2012;16:124–35.
3. Deland JT, De Asla RJ, Sung IH, et al. Posterior tibial tendon insufficiency: which ligaments are involved? Foot Ankle Int 2005;26:427–35.
4. Cromeens BP, Kirchoff CA, Patterson RM, et al. An attachment-based description of the medial collateral and spring ligament complexes. Foot Ankle Int 2015;36: 710–21.
5. Acevedo J, Vora A. Anatomical reconstruction of the spring ligament complex "Internal Brace" augmentation. Foot Ankle Spec 2013;6(6):441–5.
6. Choi K, Lee S, Otis JC, et al. Anatomical reconstruction of the spring ligament using peroneus longus tendon graft. Foot Ankle Int 2003;24(5):430–6.
7. Palmanovich E, Shabat S, Brin YS, et al. Anatomic reconstruction technique for a plantar calcaneonavicular (Spring) ligament tear. J Foot Ankle Surg 2015;54(6): 1124–6.
8. Mousavian A, Orapin J, Chinanuvathana A, et al. Anatomic spring ligament and posterior tibial tendon reconstruction: new concept of double bundle PTT and a novel technique for spring ligament. Arch Bone Jt Surg 2017; 5(3):201–5.
9. Nery C, Lemos AC, Raduan F, et al. Combined spring and deltoid ligament repair in adult-acquired flatfoot. Foot Ankle Int 2018;39(8):903–7.
10. Ryssman DB, Jang CL. Reconstruction of the spring ligament with a posterior tibial tendon autograft: technique tip. Foot Ankle Int 2017;38(4):452–6.
11. Aynardi MC, Saloky K, Roush EP, et al. Biomechanical evaluation of spring ligament augmentation with the fibertape device in a cadaveric flatfoot model. Foot Ankle Int 2019;40(5):596–602.
12. Johnson KA, Strom DE. Tibialis posterior tendon dysfunction. Clin Orthop Relat Res 1989;239:196–206.
13. Bluman EM, Title CI, Myerson MS. Posterior tibial tendon rupture: a refined classification system. Foot Ankle Clin 2007;12:233–49, v.
14. Davis WH, Sobel M, DiCarlo EF, et al. Gross, histological, and microvascular anatomy and biomechanical testing of the spring ligament complex. Foot Ankle Int 1996;17:95–102.

15. Williams BR, Ellis SJ, Deyer TW, et al. Reconstruction of the spring ligament using peroneus longus tendon autograft. Foot Ankle Int 2010;31:567–78.
16. Xu C, Li MQ, Wang C, et al. Nonanatomic versus anatomic techniques in spring ligament reconstruction: biomechanical assessment via a finite element model. J Ortho Surg Res 2019;14:114–25.
17. Myerson MS, Kadakia AR. Reconstructive foot and ankle surgery management. Philadelphia (PA): Elsevier Saunders; 2005.

A Critical Biomechanical Evaluation of Foot and Ankle Soft Tissue Repair

Sara Mateen, DPM[a], Laura E. Sansosti, DPM, FACFAS[b], Andrew J. Meyr, DPM, FACFAS[b],*

KEYWORDS

- Mechanical testing • ATFL • Talocalcaneonavicular • Plantar metatarsophalangeal
- Tendon repair • Ligamentous repair

KEY POINTS

- To understand the normal biomechanical forces extending through lower extremity soft tissue structures during physiologic function.
- To understand the biomechanical evaluation of repair techniques with mechanical testing.
- To recognize common limitations in the mechanical testing literature.
- To appreciate the difference between statistically significant and clinically significant differences in the biomechanical testing literature.

INTRODUCTION

History has demonstrated that, on balance, Sir Isaac Newton was full of it. An isolated eccentric who spent much of his time considering alchemy, the occult and doomsday prophecies, his initially groundbreaking discourses about "gravity" as an invisible and intangible force have long been demonstrated inaccurate by Albert Einstein and future generations of physicists.[1–8] Despite this, it is difficult to critically analyze the medical literature with respect to the biomechanical properties of lower extremity soft tissue repair without first understanding the unit of force for which he serves as an eponym:

- A "Newton (N)" is defined as the force required to accelerate 1 kg mass at a rate of 1 m/s^2, and
- A "Newton meter (Nm)" is a measurement of torque resulting from 1 N force applied to a 1-m moment arm.

[a] Temple University Hospital Podiatric Surgical Residency Program, Philadelphia, PA, USA;
[b] Department of Podiatric Surgery, Temple University School of Podiatric Medicine, Philadelphia, PA, USA
* Corresponding author. TUSPM Department of Surgery, 148 North 8th Street, Philadelphia, PA 19107.
E-mail address: ajmeyr@gmail.com

Clin Podiatr Med Surg 39 (2022) 521–533
https://doi.org/10.1016/j.cpm.2022.02.011
0891-8422/22/© 2022 Elsevier Inc. All rights reserved.

podiatric.theclinics.com

Although these serve as among the most frequently cited outcome measures in mechanical testing investigations, they are neither easily conceptualized nor readily applicable in terms of clinical evaluation.

With that said, however, any foot and ankle surgeon is able to develop a better understanding of these units without having to dive too deeply into the principles of physics. In fact, it is not much more complicated than the more familiar formula: pressure = force/area. Put simply, higher forces and smaller areas lead to increased pressure. The Newton unit of force is somewhat more complex in that it involves the extra dimensions of speed and distance, but the general concept is the same. Higher weights, faster speeds, and greater distances of structure contraction/extension all lead to higher force when considering the Newton. The inherent value of the unit is that it is a more dynamic and responsive measure of force, and of course the foot and ankle is a very dynamic functional anatomic area with varying forces exerted through numerous anatomic structures and in a variety of clinical situations.

The objective of this review is to provide a practical critical assessment of the literature with respect to soft tissue repair techniques in the foot and ankle. We will first review the typical forces expected through anatomic structures during their normal function, and then use this as a guide to evaluate reconstruction techniques and protocols. We hope that this will also further allow critical readers to interpret the distinction between statistically significant and clinically significant differences in the literature. For example, statistically significant differences that would not be expected to affect medical decision-making might be argued to be of little clinical value. The specific anatomic structures of the Achilles tendon, anterior tibiofibular ligament, plantar metatarsophalangeal ligament (plantar plate or plantar pad), and calcaneonavicular ligament (spring ligament) will be reviewed.

ACHILLES TENDON

The Achilles tendon almost certainly represents the lion's share of the published literature with respect to the mechanical testing analysis of lower extremity soft tissue reconstruction, and we have hopefully progressed far beyond Hippocrates' description of "this tendon, if bruised or cut, causes the most acute fevers, induces choking, deranges the mind and at length brings death".[9] Generally considered the strongest and thickest tendon in the body, the length ranges between 11 and 26 cm with a width of 4.5 to 8.6 cm.[9,10] It is comprised primarily of type 1 collagen; however, type 3 collagen is more commonly found following rupture or injury.[9] Along the tendon's length, the fibers spiral up to 90°. This might contribute to increased strength, decreased buckling, and less deformation.[9,11] The longitudinally oriented fibers also allow for significant weight-bearing and physiologic stress.

The calcaneal insertion site of the tendon represents a relatively small footprint, only about 10% of the tendon itself, but its microstructural arrangement and properties allow for maximum attachment, an increased moment arm with smooth function, and dispersion of about 2 KN of force.[12] This capability is in large part due to the off-axis orientation of the fibers and a mineral concentration of up to 50%. The collagen fibers disperse stress locally, and mineralization increases stiffness to the area, which provides coordinated protection to the insertion and transfers stress to the tendon proper.[12]

A fair amount is known about the physiologic stresses that occur through this tendon during normal function. Forces of approximately 3 KN have been reported during maximal isometric contractions, 2.6 KN during slow walking, 1 KN during cycling, and as high as 9 KN while running. This equates to approximately 12.5 times body weight or 11 KN/cm^2 when considering the cross-sectional area of the tendon.[9,10,13,14] Repetitive hopping can produce peak loads of 3.8 KN, unilateral hopping up to 5 KN, and squat jumping to 2.2 KN.[9,10,13] Ultrasonographic studies have demonstrated that maximal tendon forces range between 200 and 3800N, elongation values from 2 to 24 mm, Young modulus between 0.3 and 1.4 GPa, and stiffness of 17 to 760 N/mm.[10]

From a biomechanical perspective, the gastroc-soleus complex and Achilles tendon serve many purposes.[11] During the contact period of the gait cycle, it works to decelerate internal tibial rotation, and similarly during midstance, it decelerates anterior tibial advancement. It further acts to plantarflex the ankle joint to initiate heel off. Weakness or tightness of the complex might result in imbalances or gait cycle abnormalities, which in turn can lead to numerous ankle and foot pathologic conditions.[11] It is of course also one of the most prone tendons to rupture, largely in part due to the forces it is subject to and the relative paucity of blood supply to what has traditionally been referred to as the watershed region.[11] The incidence of Achilles tendon rupture has been reported across the literature as approximately 9.9 to 40 per 100,000 annually.[10,15] Tendons can typically stretch up to 4% before sustaining damage, but past this 4% threshold the collagen cross-links are disrupted and beyond 8% macroscopic rupture occurs.[9–11]

Backer and colleagues performed a review on 100 articles pertaining to Achilles tendon rupture and evaluated strength measurements following rupture healing.[15] Significant variability was noted with measurement style, patient positioning, angular velocity, repetitive measurements, and the use of warm-up sessions before obtaining outcomes. Results also varied across studies in terms of the reported unit of force versus direct percent comparisons to the unaffected limb. The authors concluded there is a lack of consensus on the optimal means of assessing strength following rupture. This is obviously important to consider as one views and interprets the published literature.

Sadoghi and colleagues performed a systematic review generally representative of the broader literature pertaining to initial strength analyses following end-to-end Achilles tendon repairs.[16] Eleven studies were incorporated into the analysis, and several different repair techniques were assessed including the familiar Krackow, Kessler, Bunnell, Ma-Griffith, triple bundle, and giftbox suture repairs among others. Reported tensile strengths ranged from 81 to 453 N with a mean of 222.7 N. The triple bundle technique had the highest tensile strength at 453 N, followed by the Bunnell (217.2 N), Krackow (172.7 N), giftbox (168 N), Kessler (167.7 N), and Ma-Griffith (149.5 N). Importantly, despite these apparent differences, the authors concluded that the variability in study design, sample size, and measurement techniques rendered a formal conclusion on construct superiority unfeasible.

With that said, this study provides a good example of a discussion of the difference between a statistically significant and clinically significant result. Although a statistically significant difference might easily be demonstrated between the triple bundle and Ma-Griffith techniques (453 N vs 149.5 N), for example, both groups would be expected to fail if the patient engaged in unprotected walking in the immediate postoperative period.[9,10,13,14] It is therefore reasonable to question if this statistically significant difference has any clinical significance if it does not affect postoperative medical decision-making.[14] All the described techniques would be expected to require immediate postoperative protected immobilization. A clinically significant difference, however, might be argued to be one that would allow for a faster functional recovery or change in prescribed postoperative rehabilitation protocols.

Several investigations have been published examining and comparing different end-to-end tendon repair techniques, but it seems fair to conclude that most constructs produce results with failure occurring in the ballpark of several hundred Newtons.[17–25] Even with graft augmentation, the highest observed mean load to failure we observed was 821 N.[20] Certainly, some techniques are likely to be "stronger" than the others, but the literature shows a theme of our ability to perform an end-to-end repair that is likely able to withstand forces that occur with nonweight-bearing range of motion, but that are likely to fail with unprotected weight-bearing mobilization.[9,10,13,14] Similar results are also observed when one considers tendon-to-bone repair and reattachment techniques.[14,26–35]

ANTERIOR TALOFIBULAR LIGAMENT

Injury to the lateral ankle ligaments also represents a commonly encountered pathologic condition and target for surgical repair. This most frequently occurs in inverted and plantarflexed positions with damage to the anterior talofibular ligament (ATFL) alone or in combination with the calcaneofibular ligament.[36]

Several investigations have provided insight into the normal expected forces through the ATFL. St. Pierre and colleagues found a mean tensile strength at failure of 206 N (range 58–556 N) with an equal distribution of the failure, occurring within the midsubstance of the ligament and at the talar insertion.[37] Viens and colleagues found an ultimate load to failure at 154 $\pm$ 63.7 N with a stiffness of 14.5 $\pm$ 4.4 N/mm in intact ATFL specimens.[38] Similarly, Waldrop and colleagues noted an ultimate failure load of 160.9 $\pm$ 72.2 N and a stiffness of 12.4 $\pm$ 4.1 N/mm in intact specimens.[39] Moreover, Tohyama and colleagues reported that 30 N of force should be applied during the anterior drawer testing to achieve a sufficient examination; otherwise, the amount of displacement required for the diagnosis of ankle instability might not occur.[40–42] These highlight another relative limitation of the mechanical testing literature in that protocols are only available with cadaveric methodology. In vivo measurement and testing to failure are not possible.

When considering the biomechanical strength of differing fixation options for the ATFL, it is important to consider anatomic versus nonanatomic restoration, with or without supplemental augmentation.[43] A cadaveric study performed by Shoji and colleagues evaluated cadaveric specimens in terms of intact ATFL, injured ATFL, anatomic repair of the ATFL, and nonanatomic ATFL repair, for example.[44] The overall kinematic laxity of the anatomic repair was not statistically different from an intact ATFL, and in fact internal rotation laxity was significantly increased in the nonanatomic repair at 30° and 15° of plantarflexion versus an intact ATFL. This might point toward relative advantages of augmentation in addition to primary repair.

Viens and colleagues evaluated intact ATFLs relative to repair with either suture tape augmentation alone or Brostrom with suture tape augmentation.[38] Those with suture tape augmentation alone saw an ultimate load to failure of 315.5 $\pm$ 66.8 N and stiffness of 31.4 $\pm$ 9.9 N/mm compared with 250.8 $\pm$ 122.7 N and 21.1 $\pm$ 9.1 N/mm in the Brostrom plus augmentation group and 154 $\pm$ 63.7 N with stiffness of 14.5 $\pm$ 4.4 N/mm in the intact specimens. These results might indicate that, different than the Achilles tendon, surgical techniques for the ATFL might have the ability to achieve supraphysiologic loads to failure. Conversely, however, Waldrop and colleagues compared the traditional Brostrom and suture anchor repair techniques.[39] They noted an ultimate failure load of 160.9 $\pm$ 72.2 N and a stiffness of 12.4 $\pm$ 4.1 N/mm in the intact specimens but substantially less following the Brostrum (68.2 $\pm$ 27.8 N ultimate failure load; 6 $\pm$ 2.5 N/mm stiffness), suture anchor in the fibula (79.2 $\pm$ 34.3 N ultimate failure load; 6.8 $\pm$ 2.7 N/mm stiffness), and suture anchor in the talus (75.3 $\pm$ 45.6 N ultimate failure load; 6.6$\pm$4 N/mm).

Other investigations into the use of suture anchors have found more encouraging results. Cottom and colleagues evaluated 3 different arthroscopic techniques for lateral ankle repair with suture anchors.[45] The studied groups consisted of a single-row 2-suture anchor construct, double-row 4-anchor knotless construct, and double-row 3-anchor construct. Load to failure was observed at a mean of 156.43 ± 30.39 N, 206.62 ± 55.62 N, and 246.82 ± 82.37 N, with a statistically significant difference observed between the 2-anchor and 3-anchor constructs. These all seem to be more comparable to the load to failure findings of intact ATFLs.[37–39] Stiffness in the Cottom and colleagues investigation was measured at a mean of 12.10 ± 5.43 N/m, 13.40 ± 7.98 N/m, and 12.55 ± 4.0 N/m, respectively.[45]

These and other results are interesting from a critical analysis standpoint and likely carry clinical significance.[46–49] Because the strength of repairs with augmented techniques seems to reach physiologic or even supraphysiologic values, it might imply the ability to accelerate postoperative rehabilitation and weight-bearing protocols in some situations.

PLANTAR PLATE

The plantar metatarsophalangeal ligament (plantar plate or plantar pad) is a cup-shaped, intra-articular covering of the inferior aspect of the metatarsophalangeal joint (MPJ).[50,51] It is continuous with the joint capsule both medially and laterally effectively creating a fibrocartilaginous socket for the metatarsal head.[50] The primary composition is type 1 collagen with fibers oriented both longitudinally and interwoven, creating a strong structure to resist compressive and tensile loads.[50] Pauwel theory of "causal histogenesis" describes this collagen fibril orientation with the direction of the greatest tension able to withstand most tensile forces and support the windlass mechanism.[52]

The plantar plate plays a significant role with respect to inherent MPJ stability.[53–55] Pathologic condition in this anatomic area nearly always involves excessive dorsal translation of the proximal phalanx. Although it is easy to conceptualize the digit as actively rotating in a relatively dorsal direction on the metatarsal head, in fact during stance and propulsion the digit is firmly and statically in contact with the weight-bearing surface while the metatarsal head is the structure that effectively "moves." It is admittedly challenging to recreate this functional movement with cadaveric mechanical testing protocols, as well as investigate an accurate physiologic construct considering the dynamic stabilization provided by the extrinsic tendons.

Bhatia and colleagues used cadaveric models to determine the anatomic restraints that counteract second MPJ dislocation.[56] About 37 ± 5.7 N of force was required to dislocate the MPJ with an intact capsule and plantar plate, whereas a mean force of 26 ± 5.32 N (range 22–34 N) was required to dislocate the second toe following division of the plantar plate and 20 ± 3.5 N (range 15–23 N) following sectioning of both the medial and lateral collateral ligaments. Division of both the plantar plate and collaterals resulted in dislocation after only 8 ± 4.74 N (range 5–10 N). Suero and colleagues measured and compared dorsal displacement of the proximal phalanx in isolation as well as in combination of sectioning the plantar plate and surrounding structures. The mean dorsal displacement of an intact MPJ was approximately 10.6 mm, but when both the plantar plate and the collateral ligaments were sectioned, there was a 63% increase in dorsal displacement.[57]

Indirect repair approaches not specifically addressing the anatomy might lead to inadequate results.[50,58,59] Highlander and colleagues reported that the Weil osteotomy without plantar plate repair had a 36% complication rate of floating toe deformity with a 15% recurrence rate.[60] This might indirectly point toward the need to address the plantar plate tear or disruption directly. Chalayon and colleagues compared intact sagittal plane stability of the lesser MPJ in terms of superior subluxation, dorsiflexion, and plantarflexion.[61] Overall, the mean stability of the lesser MPJs in terms of superior subluxation was 3.03 ± 0.93 N/mm, dorsiflexion was 2.07 ± 0.38 N/mm, and plantarflexion was 0.42 ± 0.06 N/mm. Disruption of the plantar plate significantly decreased stability by an average 23%.

Specific literature and materials testing plantar plate repair constructs are relatively limited. Finney and colleagues sought to assess 3 different suture configurations that might be used for plantar plate repairs (horizontal mattress, luggage-tag, and Mason-Allen suture techniques).[62] Specimens underwent cyclic loading followed by load to failure. No differences were observed in number of cycles leading to 2 mm of displacement (mattress: 19.2 ± 1.5; luggage-tag: 18.6 ± 2.9; Mason-Allen: 18.8 ± 2.0). Peak load to failure forces were reported as 115.53 ± 15.95 N for the horizontal mattress, 102.42 ± 19.33 N for the luggage-tag, and 89.96 ± 15.78 N for Mason-Allen techniques. This difference between the horizontal mattress and Mason-Allen techniques was found to be statistically significant. Displacement at failure was noted at 9.3±2 mm for the horizontal mattress, 8.1 ± 1.6 mm for the luggage-tag, and 7.6 ± 1.6 mm for the Mason-Allen techniques. The authors also measured stiffness of the constructs, which were 52.6 ± 2.8 N/mm, 50.3 ± 10.5 N/mm, and 53.9 ± 4.9 N/mm, respectively. Neither displacement nor stiffness between constructs was found to be statistically significant.

Although the horizontal mattress seemed to be superior in terms of load to failure in the Finney and colleagues study, the constructs performed similarly across other studied parameters and the clinical significance of a 25 N difference in this location is unclear.[62] This might be particularly true as the ~90 N peak load to failure observed with the Mason-Allen technique could be considered supraphysiologic when considering the Bhatia and colleagues findings of 38 N for an intact joint.[56] One should certainly be careful directly comparing the results from 2 different studies implementing 2 different mechanical testing protocols, but the Finney and colleagues results seem to indicate that all repair techniques effectively doubled the "normal" load to failure observed in the intact joints of the Bhatia and colleagues investigation.[56,62]

SPRING LIGAMENT

Another soft tissue structure providing static support is the plantar calcaneonavicular ligament. More commonly referred to as the spring ligament complex (SLC), it is a thick triangular structure composed of at least 2 distinct ligamentous bands primarily connecting the sustentaculum tali of the calcaneus to the medial aspects of the navicular.[63–65] The superomedial calcaneonavicular ligament is a fibrocartilaginous band with collagen orientation able to withstand repetitive loads, whereas the inferomedial calcaneonavicular ligament contains organized longitudinal fibers able to resist tensile forces.[63] Although there is no direct attachment to the talus, this complex is in close anatomic proximity to the medial and plantar aspects of the talonavicular joint. This, in combination with the deltoid ligament, supports the head of the talus, provides static stability to the talar head and the talonavicular joint, supports the medial longitudinal arch, and provides kinetic coupling between the forefoot and the hindfoot.[63,66–69]

This has been an area of contemporary interest with respect to the diagnosis and treatment of posterior tibial tendon dysfunction (PTTD) and peritalar subluxation. Tears or attenuation of the SLC are commonly observed in those with PTTD, and

Table 1
Summative findings of biomechanics of lower extremity soft tissue procedures

Anatomic Area	Expected Physiologic Forces	Reviewed Repair Constructs	Conclusion?
Achilles tendon	Substantial variation is noted in expected physiologic forces depending on the specific activity[9,10,13,14]	Most repair techniques noted to fail at >**100 N** and <**1000 N**[14–16]	Reviewed repair constructs seem to range from supraphysiologic when considering nonweight-bearing range of motion, but infraphysiologic when considering weight-bearing activity
ATFL	Mean loads to ligament failure observed to range between **154** and **206N** in cadaveric methodologies[37–39]	Mean loads to failure observed to range between **68 N** and**315 N** in cadaveric methodologies examining multiple repair techniques[38,39]	Reviewed repair constructs seem to range from infraphysiologic to supraphysiologic
Plantar plate (plantar metatarsophalangeal ligament)	**37 ± 5.7 N** found to dislocate the second MPJ in a cadaveric methodology with an intact joint capsule and plantar plate[56]	Mean loads to failure observed to range between **90 N** and**116 N** in a cadaveric methodologies examining 3 different repair techniques[62]	Reviewed repair constructs seem supraphysiologic
Spring ligament (plantar calcaneonavicular ligament)	A mathematical model theorized approximate forces of **50 N** with 2-foot stance and **82 N** with single limb stance[80]	No direct analyses reviewed	This likely represents an interesting avenue for future investigation

some have proposed that this is likely the structure that fails first within the pathogenesis of peritalar subluxation, and its primary repair in flatfoot reconstructive surgeries has become more commonplace.[70–79]

With that said, it is a structure that is difficult to evaluate in isolation, both with respect to normal function and following surgical reconstruction. Cheung and colleagues concluded that force loaded on the SLC was approximately 50 N during 2-foot balance and gait, and that this increases to 82 N with single limb stance.[80] Huang and colleagues performed a cadaveric study to assess the significance of the plantar fascia, long and short plantar ligaments, and the spring ligament in maintaining arch stability.[81] Specimens were loaded to 230 N, 460 N, and 690 N with sequential sectioning of the aforementioned structures in various orders. Failure occurred at 920N when all 3 structures were sectioned. The observed decrease in arch height was greatest following sectioning of the plantar fascia regardless of order of release. This was followed by the plantar ligaments and, finally, the spring ligament. Stiffness decreased by 25%, 10%, and 2% following sectioning of the plantar fascia, plantar ligaments, and spring ligament, respectively.

Cifuentes-De la Portilla and colleagues evaluated different flatfoot arthrodesis and visualized the different stresses on osseous and cartilaginous structures following each procedure.[82–84] The highest stresses occurred at the navicular and the authors largely contributed this to the spring ligament. In an earlier study by the same authors, the biomechanical forces of each isolated joint following rearfoot arthrodesis were assessed. The talonavicular joint arthrodesis generated a significant stress reduction in comparison to the subtalar joint fusion, indirectly providing evidence to the importance of this anatomic area and supporting structures.[83]

Biomechanical testing of the SLC represents an interesting avenue for future investigations because very few have attempted this. However, Aynardi and colleagues did find significant difference in failure properties between traditional spring ligament repair and repair augmented with FiberTape[85] (**Table 1**).

CLINICS CARE POINTS

- The triple bundle technique for end to end repair of the Achilles tendon offers the highest tensile strength at 453 N compared to other techniques such as a the Bunnell, Krackow, Kessler, gift box, and Ma-Griffith.
- However, it is important to differentiate between statistically significance and clinical significance as it pertains to post-operative protocol with Achilles tendon repair.
- When considering ATFL repair, it is important to identify and consider anatomic versus nonanatomic repair and also with and without augmentation with allograft.
- Suture anchors in ATFL repair have had encouraging results and likely carry clinical significance.
- The plantar plate plays a significant role in MPJ stability along with the capsule and collateral ligaments.
- It is important to consider indirect versus direct repair of the plantar plate as it can affect recurrence rate.
- The spring ligament in combination with the deltoid ligament provide static stability to the talar head and talonavicular joint.
- Attenutation to this structure can result in the pathogenesis of peritalar subluxation and restoration of this ligament can aid in flatfoot reconstruction.

DISCLOSURE

All authors have no financial disclosures to report.

REFERENCES

1. Newton I. Observations upon the prophecies of Daniel, and the apocalypse of St. John. Glascow (United Kingdom): Good Press; 2019. p. 1–105.
2. Dry S. The Newton papers: the strange and true odyssey of Isaac Newton's manuscripts. Cary (NC): Oxford University Press; 2014.
3. Chambers J. The metaphysical world of Isaac Newton: alchemy, prophecy, and the search for lost knowledge. Merrimac (MA): Destiny Books; 2018. p. 1–408.
4. Gates J, Pelletier C. Proving Einstein right: the Daring expeditions that changed how we look at the universe. New York: PublicAffairs; 2019.
5. Stanley M. Einstein's war: how relativity triumphed amid the vicious nationalism of world war 1. London (United Kingdom): Penguin Audio; 2019.
6. Robinson A. The last man who knew everything: Thomas young, the anonymous polymath who proved Newton wrong, explained how we see, cured the sick, and deciphered the Rosetta stone, among other feats of genius. Serbia: Pi Press; 2005. p. 1–304.
7. Bauer LA. Resume of observations concerning the solar eclipse of May 29, 1919, and the Einstein effect. Science 1920;51:301–11.
8. Chant CA. Einstein displacement on the plates taken by the Canadian party at the Australian eclipse. Science 1923;57:469.
9. Doral NM, Alam M, Bozkurt M, et al. Functional anatomy of the Achilles tendon. Knee Surg Sports Traumatol Arthrosc 2010;18:638–43.
10. Winnicki K, Ochala-Klos A, Rutowicz B, et al. Functional anatomy, histology and biomechanics of the human Achilles tendon – a comprehensive review. Ann Anat 2020;229:151461.
11. Dayton P. Anatomic, vascular, and mechanical overview of the Achilles tendon. Clin Podiatr Med Surg 2017;34:107–13.
12. Sadeghi S, Taghizadeh H. Microstructural modeling of Achilles tendon biomechanics focusing on bone insertion site. Med Eng Phys 2020;78:48–54.
13. Joseph MF, Lillie KR, Bergeron DJ, et al. Achilles tendon biomechanics in response to acute intense exercise. J Strength Cond Res 2014;28:1181–6.
14. Lakey E, Kumparatana P, Moon DK, et al. Biomechanical comparison of all-soft suture anchor single-row vs double-row bridging construct for insertional Achilles tendinopathy. Foot Ankle Int 2020;42:215–23.
15. Backer HC, Yenchak AJ, Trofa DP, et al. Strength measurement after Achilles tendon repair. Foot Ankle Spec 2019;12:471–9.
16. Sadoghi P, Rosso C, Valderrabano V, et al. Initial Achilles tendon repair strength-synthesized biomechanical data from 196 cadaver repairs. Int Orthop 2012;36:1947–51.
17. Wu Z, Hua Y, Li H, et al. Biomechanical comparison of three methods for distal Achilles tendon reconstruction. Knee Surg Sports Traumatol Arthrosc 2015;23:3756–60.
18. Tian J, Rui R, Xu Y, et al. Achilles tendon rupture repair: biomechanical comparison of the locking block modified Krackow technique and the Giftbox technique. Injury 2020;51:559–64.
19. Tian J, Rui Y, Xu Y, et al. A biomechanical comparison of Achilles tendon suture repair techniques: locking block modified Krackow, Kessler, and percutaneous

Achilles repair system with early rehabilitation program in vitro bovine model. Arch Orthop Trauma Surg 2020;140:1775–82.

20. Magnussen RA, Glisson RR, Moorman CT. Augmentation of Achilles tendon repair with extracellular matrix xenograft. Am J Sports Med 2011;39(7):1522–7.

21. Wagner P, Wagner E, Lopez M, et al. Proximal and distal failure site analysis in percutaneous Achilles tendon rupture repair. Foot Ankle Int 2019;40:1424–9.

22. McCoy BW, Haddad SL. The strength of Achilles tendon repair: a comparison of three suture techniques in human cadaver tendons. Foot Ankle Int 2010;31:701–5.

23. Carmont MR, Kuiper JH, Silbernagel KG, et al. Tendon end separation with loading in an Achilles tendon repair model: comparison of non-absorbable vs. absorbable sutures. J Exp Orthop 2017;4:26.

24. Nguyen TP, Keyt LK, Herfat S, et al. Biomechanical study of a multifilament stainless steel cable crimp system versus a multistrand ultra-high molecular weight polyethylene polyester suture Krackow technique for Achilles tendon rupture repair. J Foot Ankle Surg 2020;59:86–90.

25. Cottom JM, Baker JS, Richardson PE, et al. Evaluation of a new knotless suture anchor repair in acute Achilles tendon ruptures: a biomechanical comparison of three techniques. J Foot Ankle Surg 2017;56:423–7.

26. Yammine K, Assi C. Efficacy of repair techniques of the Achilles tendon: a meta-analysis of human cadaveric biomechanical studies. Foot 2017;30:13–20.

27. Leung KS, Chong WS, Chow DHK, et al. A comparative study on the biomechanical and histological properties of bone-to-bone, bone-to-tendon, and tendon-to-tendon healing. An Achilles tendon-calcaneus model in goats. Am J Sports Med 2015;43(6):1413–21.

28. Boin MA, Dorweiler MA, McMellen CJ, et al. Suture-only repair versus suture anchor-augmented repair for Achilles tendon ruptures with a short distal stump. Orthop J Sports Med 2017;5(1). 2325967116678722.

29. Beitzel K, Mazzocca AD, Obopilwe E, et al. Biomechanical properties of double- and single-row suture anchor repair for surgical treatment of insertional Achilles tendinopathy. Am J Sports Med 2013;41(7):1642–8.

30. Awogni D, Chauvette G, Lemieux ML, et al. Button fixation technique for Achilles tendon reinsertion: a biomechanical study. J Foot Ankle Surg 2014;53:141–6.

31. Pilson H, Brown P, Stitzel J, et al. Single-row versus double-row repair of the distal Achilles tendon: a biomechanical comparison. J Foot Ankle Surg 2012;51:762–6.

32. Cox JT, Shorten PL, Gould GC, et al. Knotted versus knotless suture bridge repair of the Achilles tendon insertion. Am J Sports Med 2014;42(11):2727–33.

33. Fanter NJ, Davis EW, Baker CL. Fixation of the Achilles tendon insertion using suture button technology. Am J Sports Med 2012;40(9):2085–91.

34. Drakos MC, Gott M, Karnovsky SC, et al. Biomechanical analysis of suture anchor vs tenodesis screw for FHL transfer. Foot Ankle Int 2017;38(7):797–801.

35. Hembree WC, Tsai MA, Parks BG, et al. Comparison of suture-based anchors and traditional bioabsorbable anchors in foot and ankle surgery. J Foot Ankle Surg 2017;56:3–7.

36. McKeon BP, Heming JF, Fulkerson J, et al. The Krackow stitch: a biomechanical evaluation of changing the number of loops versus the number of sutures. Arthroscopy 2006;22:33–7.

37. St. Pierre RK, Rosen J, Whitesides TE, et al. The tensile strength of the anterior talofibular ligament. Foot Ankle 1983;4:83–5.

38. Viens NA, Wijdicks CA, Campbell KJ, et al. Anterior talofibular ligament ruptures, part 1: biomechanical comparison of augmented Broström repair techniques with the intact anterior talofibular ligament. Am J Sports Med 2014;42:405–11.
39. Waldrop NE 3rd, Wijdicks CA, Jansson KS, et al. Anatomic suture anchor versus the Brostrom technique for anterior talofibular ligament repair: a biomechanical comparison. Am J Sports Med 2012;40:2590–6.
40. Tohyama H, Yasuda K, Ohkoshi Y, et al. Anterior drawer test for acute anterior talofibular ligament injuries of the ankle. How much load should be applied during the test? Am J Sports Med 2003;31:226–32.
41. Fujii T, Luo ZP, Kitaoka HB, et al. The manual stress test may not be sufficient to differentiate ankle ligament injuries. Clin Biomech 2000;15:619–23.
42. Phisitkul P, Chaichankul C, Sripongsai R, et al. Accuracy of anterolateral drawer test in lateral ankle instability: a cadaveric study. Foot Ankle Int 2009;30:690–5.
43. Lohrer H, Bonsignore G, Dorn-Lange N, et al. Stabilizing lateral ankle instability by suture tape - a cadaver study. J Orthop Surg Res 2019;14:175.
44. Shoji H, Teramoto A, Sakakibara Y, et al. Kinematics and laxity of the ankle joint in anatomic and nonanatomic anterior talofibular ligament repair: a biomechanical cadaveric study. Am J Sports Med 2019;47:667–73.
45. Cottom JM, Baker JS, Richardson PE, et al. A biomechanical comparison of 3 different arthroscopic lateral ankle stabilization techniques in 36 cadaveric ankles. J Foot Ankle Surg 2016;55:1229–33.
46. Li H, Zhao Y, Hua Y, et al. Knotless anchor repair produced similarly favourable outcomes as knot anchor repair for anterior talofibular ligament repair. Knee Surg Sports Traumatol Arthrosc 2020;28:3987–93.
47. Jung HG, Kim TH, Park JY, et al. Anatomic reconstruction of the anterior talofibular and calcaneofibular ligaments using a semitendinosus tendon allograft and interference screws. Knee Surg Sports Traumatol Arthrosc 2012;20:1432–7.
48. Choi HJ, Kim DW, Park JS. Modified Broström procedure using distal fibular periosteal flap augmentation vs anatomic reconstruction using a free tendon allograft in patients who are not candidates for standard repair. Foot Ankle Int 2017;38:1207–14.
49. Giza E, Shin EC, Wong SE, et al. Arthroscopic suture anchor repair of the lateral ligament ankle complex. Am J Sports Med 2013;41:2567–72.
50. Camasta C. Plantar plate repair of the second metatarsophalangeal joint. In: Southerland JT, Boberg JS, Downey MS, et al, editors. McGlamry's comprehensive textbook of foot and ankle surgery. 4th Edition. Philadelphia (PA): Lippincott Williams & Wilkins; 2013. p. 187–201.
51. Maas NM, van der Grinten M, Bramer WM, et al. Metatarsophalangeal joint stability: a systematic review on the plantar plate of the lesser toes. J Foot Ankle Res 2016;9:32.
52. Petersen W, Tillmann B. Structure and vascularization of the cruciate ligaments of the human knee joint. Anat Embryol (Berl) 1999;200:325–34.
53. Fleischer AE, Hshieh S, Crews RT, et al. Association between second metatarsal length and forefoot loading under the second metatarsophalangeal joint. Foot Ankle Int 2018;39:560–7.
54. Landorf KB, Ackland CA, Bonanno DR, et al. Effects of metatarsal domes on plantar pressures in older people with a history of forefoot pain. J Foot Ankle Res 2020;13:18.
55. Coughlin MJ. Second metatarsophalangeal joint instability in the athlete. Foot Ankle 1993;14:309–19.

56. Bhatia D, Myerson MS, Curtis MJ, et al. Anatomical restraints to dislocation of the second metatarsophalangeal joint and assessment of a repair technique. J Bone Joint Surg Am 1994;76:1371–5.

57. Suero EM, Meyers KN, Bohne WH. Stability of the metatarsophalangeal joint of the lesser toes: a cadaveric study. J Orthop Res 2012;30:1995–8.

58. Ford LA, Collins KB, Christensen JC. Stabilization of the subluxed second metatarsophalangeal joint: flexor tendon transfer versus primary repair of the plantar plate. J Foot Ankle Surg 1998;37:217–22.

59. Sung W. Technique using interference fixation repair for plantar plate ligament disruption of lesser metatarsophalangeal joints. J Foot Ankle Surg 2015;54:508–12.

60. Highlander P, VonHerbulis E, Gonzalez A, et al. Complications of the Weil osteotomy. Foot Ankle Spec 2011;4:165–70.

61. Chalayon O, Chertman C, Guss AD, et al. Role of plantar plate and surgical reconstruction techniques on static stability of lesser metatarsophalangeal joints: a biomechanical study. Foot Ankle Int 2013;34:1436–42.

62. Finney FT, Lee S, Scott J, et al. Biomechanical evaluation of suture configurations in lesser toe plantar plate repairs. Foot Ankle Int 2018;39:836–42.

63. Rule J, Yao L, Seeger LL. Spring ligament of the ankle: normal MR anatomy. Am J Roentgenol 1993;161:1241–4.

64. Lin YC, Kwon JY, Ghorbanhoseini M, et al. The hindfoot arch: what role does the imager play? Radiol Clin North Am 2016;54:951–68.

65. Davis WH, Sobel M, DiCarlo EF, et al. Gross, histological, and microvascular anatomy and biomechanical testing of the spring ligament complex. Foot Ankle Int 1996;17:95–102.

66. Van Boerum DH, Sangeorzan BJ. Biomechanics and pathophysiology of flat foot. Foot Ankle Clin 2003;8:419–30.

67. Reeck J, Felten N, McCormack AP, et al. Support of the talus: a biomechanical investigation of the contributions of the talonavicular and talocalcaneal joints, and the superomedial calcaneonavicular ligament. Foot Ankle Int 1998;19(10):674–82.

68. Masaragian HJ, Massetti S, Perin F, et al. Flatfoot deformity due to isolated spring ligament injury. J Foot Ankle Surg 2020;59:469–78.

69. Bastias GF, Dalmau-Pastor M, Astudillo C, et al. Spring ligament instability. Foot Ankle Clin 2018;23:659–78.

70. Deland JT, de Asla RJ, Sung IH, et al. Posterior tibial tendon insufficiency: which ligaments are involved? Foot Ankle Int 2005;26:427–35.

71. Kelly M, Masqoodi N, Vasconcellos D, et al. Spring ligament tear decreases static stability of the ankle joint. Clin Biomech 2019;61:79–83.

72. Myerson MS, Thordarson DB, Johnson JE, et al. Classification and nomenclature: progressive collapsing foot deformity. Foot Ankle Int 2020;41:1271–6.

73. Thordarson DB, Schmotzer H, Chon J, et al. Dynamic support of the human longitudinal arch. A biomechanical evaluation. Clin Orthop Relat Res 1995;316:165–72.

74. Thordarson DB, Schmotzer H, Chon J. Reconstruction with tenodesis in an adult flatfoot model. A biomechanical evaluation of four methods. J Bone Joint Surg Am 1995;77:1557–64.

75. Tryfonidis M, Jackson W, Mansour R, et al. Acquired adult flat foot due to isolated plantar calcaneonavicular (spring) ligament insufficiency with a normal tibialis posterior tendon. Foot Ankle Surg 2008;14:89–95.

76. Pasapula C, Devany A, Fischer NC, et al. The resistance to failure of spring ligament reconstruction. Foot (Edinb) 2017;33:29–34.
77. Pasapula C, Devany A, Magan A, et al. Neutral heel lateral push test: the first clinical examination of spring ligament integrity. Foot (Edinb) 2015;25:69–74.
78. Flores DV, Mejía Gómez C, Fernández Hernando M, et al. Adult acquired flatfoot deformity: anatomy, biomechanics, staging, and imaging findings. Radiographics 2019;39:1437–60.
79. Ellis SJ, Williams BR, Wagshul AD, et al. Deltoid ligament reconstruction with peroneus longus autograft in flatfoot deformity. Foot Ankle Int 2010;31:781–9.
80. Cheung JT, Zhang M, An KN. Effects of plantar fascia stiffness on the biomechanical responses of the ankle-foot complex. Clin Biomech 2004;19:839–46.
81. Huang CK, Kitaoka HB, An KN, et al. Biomechanical evaluation of longitudinal arch stability. Foot Ankle 1993;14:353–7.
82. Cifuentes-De la Portilla C, Pasapula C, Larrainzar-Garijo R, et al. Finite element analysis of secondary effect of midfoot fusions on the spring ligament in the management of adult acquired flatfoot. Clin Biomech 2020;76:105018.
83. Cifuentes-De la Portilla C, Larrainzar-Garijo R, Bayod J. Analysis of the main passive soft tissues associated with adult acquired flatfoot deformity development: a computational modeling approach. J Biomech 2019;84:183–90.
84. Cifuentes-De la Portilla C, Larrainzar-Garijo R, Bayod J. Analysis of biomechanical stresses caused by hindfoot joint arthrodesis in the treatment of adult acquired flatfoot deformity: a finite element study. Foot Ankle Surg 2020;26:412–20.
85. Aynardi MC, Saloky K, Roush EP, et al. Biomechanical evaluation of spring ligament augmentation with the FiberTape device in a cadaveric flatfoot model. Foot Ankle Int 2019;40:596–602.

Printed and bound by CPI Group (UK) Ltd, Croydon, CR0 4YY

03/10/2024

01040469-0016